THE EVERYTHING®

GUIDE TO
INTEGRATIVE PAIN MANAGEMENT

Dear Reader,

As I'm sure you know, having chronic pain challenges you on every level—emotionally, physically, socially, and spiritually. All too often, it can take years to find the right combination of therapies to help you find peace and comfort in the body you actually have, even if it is not working "perfectly." The trial and error can be frustrating, but the sense of mastery you gain from taking an active role in your health will be liberating, even if the symptoms don't completely go away.

One thing to remember is that your body-mind has some very powerful built-in mechanisms to help you manage pain and feel better in general. Each person's journey is different—there is no one-size-fits-all approach. But, with a little practice and the best of conventional and complementary medicine, you *can* change your pain experience, and your life, in general, for the better. You may not get rid of your symptoms completely, but you can take the reins from pain and live a life that has meaning for you—just as you are, right now—even as you continue to work toward change. Please feel free to use this book in combination with other tools you already find helpful.

Be well!

Traci Stein

Welcome to the EVERYTHING® Series!

These handy, accessible books give you all you need to tackle a difficult project, gain a new hobby, comprehend a fascinating topic, prepare for an exam, or even brush up on something you learned back in school but have since forgotten.

You can choose to read an Everything® book from cover to cover or just pick out the information you want from our four useful boxes: e-questions, e-facts, e-alerts, and e-ssentials.

We give you everything you need to know on the subject, but throw in a lot of fun stuff along the way, too.

We now have more than 400 Everything® books in print, spanning such wide-ranging categories as weddings, pregnancy, cooking, music instruction, foreign language, crafts, pets, New Age, and so much more. When you're done reading them all, you can finally say you know Everything®!

QUESTION

Answers to common questions

FACT

Important snippets of information

ALERT

Urgent warnings

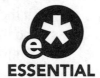

ESSENTIAL

Quick handy tips

PUBLISHER Karen Cooper

MANAGING EDITOR, EVERYTHING® SERIES Lisa Laing

COPY CHIEF Casey Ebert

ASSISTANT PRODUCTION EDITOR Alex Guarco

ACQUISITIONS EDITOR Eileen Mullan

ASSOCIATE DEVELOPMENT EDITOR Eileen Mullan

EVERYTHING® SERIES COVER DESIGNER Erin Alexander

Visit the entire Everything® series at *www.everything.com*

THE
EVERYTHING®
GUIDE TO
Integrative Pain Management

Conventional and alternative therapies for managing pain

Traci Stein, PhD, MPH

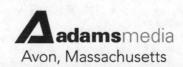
Avon, Massachusetts

To my patients, who continue to teach me so much.
And in memory of Dr. Samantha Boris Karpel, a
beautiful soul and tireless advocate for those in pain.

An Everything® Series Book.
Everything® and everything.com® are registered trademarks of F+W Media, Inc.

Published by
Adams Media, a division of F+W Media, Inc.
57 Littlefield Street, Avon, MA 02322. U.S.A.
www.adamsmedia.com

ISBN 10: 1-4405-8970-4
ISBN 13: 978-1-4405-8970-6
eISBN 10: 1-4405-8971-2
eISBN 13: 978-1-4405-8971-3

Printed in the United States of America.

10 9 8 7 6 5 4 3 2 1

Library of Congress Cataloging-in-Publication Data
Stein, Traci.
The everything guide to integrative pain management / Traci Stein, PhD, MPH.
pages cm
Includes index.
ISBN 978-1-4405-8970-6 (pb) -- ISBN 1-4405-8970-4 (pb) -- ISBN 978-1-4405-8971-3 (ebook) -- ISBN 1-4405-8971-2 (ebook)
1. Integrative medicine. 2. Chronic pain--Alternative treatment. I. Title.
R733.S74 2015
616'.0472--dc23

2015022670

Contents

Acknowledgments

My continued gratitude to those Columbia University mentors and colleagues, past and present, who have shared their wisdom, including but not limited to Dr. Nomita Sonty, Dr. Michael Weinberger, and Dr. James Dillard. Dr. Roni Beth Tower, many thanks for encouraging me to think outside the box and supporting my love for and use of mind-body therapies, especially imagery. Thanks to Judy Kurzer, LCSW, who helped me formalize my training in clinical hypnosis and who continues to provide valuable feedback and support about this, one of my favorite tools for a range of conditions. My thanks to Dr. Mehmet Oz for giving me my formal start in Integrative Medicine all those years ago. A very special thank you to my former Columbia mentor and now colleague, Dr. John Saroyan, for his friendship, encouragement, and invaluable feedback on this manuscript. And finally, to my husband Jason and our little family—Morty, Mitzi, Petie, and Sebastian—for your unwavering support, patience, and good humor.

Top Ten Things to Remember about Integrative Pain Management

1. You are the most important person on your pain management team; *you* must be the team captain.

2. You are far more than your body and how it looks, functions, or feels on any given day.

3. It's worth making healthy lifestyle changes even if you don't notice a direct impact on your pain initially.

4. Let go of comparisons to other people or to your former self!

5. All change takes place in the now.

6. Your peace of mind, acceptance of your body, and commitment to your well-being should be independent of whether other people understand what you are going through.

7. Your pain management program will evolve as you do. Your open-mindedness, curiosity, and flexibility will help you adapt your approach to your body's changing needs and abilities.

8. Sometimes the most effective tools will be the simplest, such as self-compassion, being in the present moment, having a sense of humor, and remembering to breathe.

9. There is no one right way to manage pain. The right way is the one that works best for you, respects who you are, and honors your inherent worth.

10. You *can* create a life that has meaning, despite pain.

Introduction

CHANCES ARE THAT IF you are reading this book, you have been diagnosed with one of the many conditions that fall under the heading of "chronic pain." What may have begun as a "normal" painful response to injury or illness has now persisted long after the tissue or bone has healed. Or perhaps, even more perplexing, your pain arose seemingly "out of nowhere" in the absence of any distinct trauma to your body, but rather, due to an immune issue, changes in your brain, a condition with which you were born, or a cause not yet realized, but is still painful nonetheless. And although many, many people suffer from pain that has continued long after it serves any purpose, you may very well have felt alone or frustrated in your struggle to access relief or understanding from medical providers or those close to you.

Chronic pain is the most prevalent public health problem in the United States and worldwide, affecting over 100 million American adults and an estimated 1.5 billion people on the planet. Each year, chronic pain results in the loss of hundreds of billions of dollars to the economy. And unlike many other conditions, for all intents and purposes pain is invisible and can persist despite the absence of objective "evidence" via imaging, blood work, or other diagnostic tests. Because of this invisibility, pain has unique social, interpersonal, and occupational costs. Friends, family, coworkers, and even healthcare providers who might otherwise be sympathetic to an observable medical issue may be baffled by or doubtful of a condition that is both debilitating and unseen.

If you suffer from chronic pain, you are probably already aware of the many distressing emotions, such as grief, anxiety, sadness, fear, resentment, and feelings of powerlessness associated with unremitting pain. It's also likely that pain has caused changes in your sleep quality, concentration, appetite, energy levels, sex life, or ability to fulfill aspects of your duties as a parent, partner, student, friend, or employee. You may feel overwhelmed by an increasing number of doctors' appointments and statements from loved ones that are intended to be helpful, but ultimately feel judgmental or simply unhelpful ("You just need to ignore the pain" or "I get headaches too, but I just take aspirin and get on with my day"). Depending on your insurance coverage and ability to work, you may also feel significant worry about how you will survive financially as you strive to solve the riddle of your pain.

Furthermore, pain can make it more challenging to communicate effectively with your medical team, as well as with others who are important to you. The chronic stress of being in pain may prompt you to express yourself in ways that later leave you feeling guilty or ineffective, or further strain important relationships.

As if these challenges weren't enough, having chronic pain can lead you to forget that you are, by far, *the most important member of your pain management team*, and that there is a good deal you *can* do to feel better. The good news is that by crafting an individualized program, perhaps with some of the tools mentioned in this book, you may find that you achieve a greater sense of peace and well-being than you had *even before* you were in pain. With that in mind, use this book as a starting point to expand your ideas of healing and personal wellness, practice good self-care, communicate your needs effectively, and create the healthcare team that is best suited to you. As you read about some of the therapies, you may wish to investigate them further, experiment with different healing regimens, and commit to putting yourself back in the driver's seat of your life.

CHAPTER 1

Integrative Pain Management

Having chronic pain, by definition, changes how "normal" feels. If you are in pain, how you feel physically and emotionally and how you function in daily life are different than they are for someone who does not suffer from chronic pain. For example, perhaps you suffered an injury or experienced sudden discomfort. Like most people, your first question was probably, "What's going on?"—especially if there was no clear event or injury triggering the pain. The next likely question was, "When will I feel better?" As your pain stretched on for weeks, and then months, you almost certainly worried about how you could "get back to normal" and what might happen if your normal is never what it once was.

The Experience of Pain

Regardless of the treatment plan you choose to treat your pain, it's important to have a good understanding of pain and pain-related terms. This will help you communicate more effectively with your providers, understand the particular things that make your pain worse or better, and craft the approach that is best suited to you.

FACT

It's hard to believe, but ongoing pain affects more people than cancer, heart disease, and diabetes combined. According to the American Academy of Pain Medicine, that's almost one-third of the population, or 100 million people in the United States alone!

Pain is universally described as an unpleasant physical sensation that can vary with regard to both the severity of discomfort (how much it hurts) and the degree of emotional and cognitive distress that it causes (how much it bothers you). One thing about pain that surprises many people is that regardless of the type of pain or where you experience the sensation, pain is a brain-derived phenomenon. To put it simply, without your brain interpreting the signals from your body (or, in some cases, acting on its own *despite* a lack of input from the body), you would not feel pain at all.

One thing that makes it much more difficult to cope with chronic pain is that often it exists in the absence of objective evidence (i.e., medically identifiable causes) that can be seen on X-ray, MRI, or other imaging. This issue tends to increase frustration for both patients and doctors as to how to best treat the pain. It also makes it more difficult for family and friends to "get it." The lack of an image pinpointing the cause of your pain *does not* mean it isn't real, however.

Describing Pain

There are many ways to describe the sensations that your brain files under the heading of pain. Depending on the type of pain you have, you probably find yourself using some labels more than others in an attempt to convey what you are experiencing.

The following table features the most common pain descriptors. It's worth noting the terms you use most often, and perhaps circling them or writing them down before meeting with your doctor, as this information will be useful in helping her decide which treatments might be most effective for your type of pain.

PAIN LABELS

Sharp	Stinging	Pounding
Throbbing	Intermittent	Constant
Electrical	Aching	Stabbing
Hot	Cutting	Tight
Squeezing	Crushing	Tugging
Dull	Burning	Itchy
Radiating	Severe	Mild

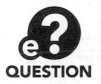

QUESTION

Pain is awful! Why do people experience it at all?
Pain, though undeniably unpleasant and often distressing, is actually essential for your survival. Congenital analgesia is a genetic disorder where one *can't* feel pain. People with this condition have more frequent and worse injuries and also die younger because they can't feel the normal pain that tells the body to avoid harm.

Acute Pain

Acute pain is a time-limited response, usually regarding injury to soft tissue or bone. You could think of acute pain as "pain with a purpose" because it indicates that something is hurting you and thus requires you to react in some way. Pain is the body's warning sign that damage has occurred or is taking place. It's a signal to pay attention and either stop doing the action that is causing the pain (such as when you touch a hot stove and your brain tells you to jerk your hand away from it), or to do something to protect yourself and guard against further injury (such as running the finger you just burned under cold water).

Acute pain lessens as the injured area heals and returns to normal. This type of pain can be caused by minor trauma (such as bumping into something), a major trauma (such as a serious accident), an illness (such as cancer, when a tumor may impinge on surrounding tissue), or result from an infection. Pain also occurs as a result of abnormal stretching of tissue (such as when a muscle is pulled or strained), too much pressure on a sensitive area (such as when you try to walk in shoes that are too tight, for too long), or when tissue is inflamed and in the process of healing. Other situations that generate pain but are not necessarily indicative of injury include muscles or organs cramping.

Acute pain often comes on suddenly (such as when you stub your toe) and is time-limited by definition. This type of pain usually lasts anywhere from a few seconds to a few weeks. Acute pain sometimes resolves as soon as the source of the pain is removed (such as when you remove the too-tight shoe). But again, acute pain has a purpose—it's one way of your body doing its job to protect you from harm and keep you safe as you heal.

Chronic Pain

Chronic pain, depending on the definition used, has lasted three to six months or more—well beyond it serving any sort of useful purpose. There are many different painful conditions—too many to list completely here, but in the table is a sampling of some you may have heard of or be experiencing yourself.

EXAMPLES OF CHRONIC PAIN CONDITIONS

Gastrointestinal (Crohn's Disease, Irritable Bowel Syndrome, Colitis, Gastroesophogeal Reflux Disease or GERD)	Headaches (Tension-Type, Migraine, Cluster)
Fibromyalgia	Dental Pain
Myofascial Pain	Temporomandibular Joint Disorder
Cancer Pain	Musculoskeletal Pain
Arthritis	Pain from Circulatory Issues
Sickle Cell Anemia	Phantom Limb Pain
Endometriosis Pain	Neuropathic Pain (Postherpetic Neuralgia, Diabetic Peripheral Neuropathy, Complex Regional Pain Syndrome)
Back Pain	Carpal Tunnel Syndrome

An Integrative Approach to Pain

Integrative medicine combines conventional medical treatments, such as drugs, surgery, or medical devices, with therapies that fall under the headings "complementary" (used with conventional medicine) or "alternative." Mind-body approaches, such as meditation, hypnosis, and relaxation training; movement-based therapies, such as yoga and tai chi; nutritional approaches and dietary supplements; energy therapies, such as Reiki; and other systems of healing that fall outside Western medicine, can all be considered complementary and alternative medicine (CAM). Many of these can be thoughtfully integrated with your medical treatment to help you manage pain and feel better overall—body, mind, and spirit.

In these pages, you will see "integrative" used to refer to the broad approach just described. Sometimes the term CAM will be used to indicate the use of a nonmedical treatment, whether on its own or as part of an integrative program. Understand that this book, rather than placing one type of therapy over any other for managing pain, encourages you to enhance your knowledge of treatments that may help in some way and create the plan that works best for you.

The National Center for Complementary and Integrative Health (NCCIH; formerly the National Center for Complementary and Alternative Medicine) is the U.S. government's lead agency for conducting research into the use and effectiveness of CAM therapies. Much has been learned about CAM therapies and trends since the center's creation in 1998. In fact, it's estimated that more than one-third of adults and 12 percent of children use CAM in a given year. This amounts to about $34 billion annually that Americans spend, largely out of pocket, for therapies like massage, acupuncture, yoga, chiropractic, and others. When including dietary supplement use, the percentage of adults increases to over 50 percent. Many, many of these consumers are using CAM to treat chronic pain conditions such as back pain, arthritis, and headaches.

Here is a list of the most popular CAM therapies used by adults, according to the National Health Interview Survey:

MOST POPULAR CAM THERAPIES

Omega 3 Supplements/ Fish Oil	Glucosamine	Echinacea	Flaxseed
Ginseng	Combination Herbal Pills	Gingko Biloba	Chondroitin
Garlic	Coenzyme Q10	Deep Breathing	Chiropractic and Osteopathy
Massage	Yoga	Diet-Based Therapies	Progressive Relaxation
Guided Imagery	Homeopathic Treatments		

FACT

Given that roughly 100 million U.S. adults have used at least one CAM therapy in the past year, the odds that *you* have used a CAM therapy, even if you weren't thinking of it as such, are actually pretty good!

There are many more CAM therapies than the ones listed, or that can be covered in this book, but in these pages you will find overviews of those therapies that have several things in common:

- Some evidence of benefit for managing pain
- Low risk of undesirable effects
- In many cases, can be combined easily with the conventional approaches you are already using
- Lead to increased feelings of calm and relaxation

Although the term "integrative" primarily will be used throughout the remainder of this book in order to be as inclusive and current as possible, you should keep in mind that your personal journey may at different points be completely conventional, very integrative, or solely alternative, depending on what you discover is most helpful for you at a particular time. Your medical team is the best resource for understanding the potential role of conventional therapies, and hopefully will continue to be a resource you can consult even if your treatment plan shifts to something more CAM in nature. As you feel increasing symptom relief, your interactions with your medical team may shift to a greater emphasis on periodic monitoring of your medical condition rather than on interventions. Regardless of the approach you choose, you are encouraged to keep your medical team in the loop and notify them of any changes in your symptoms or functioning.

FACT

Both the American College of Physicians and the American Pain Society state that nondrug approaches should be considered in patients who do not improve with self-care. Some of the recommendations, such as exercise therapy and cognitive-behavioral therapy, are conventional. Other therapies are considered CAM and include acupuncture, massage therapy, spinal manipulation, and progressive relaxation.

Creating the Approach that Is Right for You

The aim of an integrative approach is to assist you in developing the regimen that feels most helpful to you, enables you to feel greater mastery over your healthcare plan, utilizes therapies that are enjoyable to you in some way, is consistent with your personal preferences and beliefs with regard to healing, and honors where you are in your healing journey at a given point in time. Specific to the last point, you may notice that you continue to fine tune or update your regimen as your physical health, general well-being, finances, life circumstances, or openness to new therapies changes over time.

ESSENTIAL

Because managing pain and other physical and emotional symptoms can feel overwhelming, you may find yourself wishing someone else could do it for you. It's a totally understandable desire, *but you are the only person who can do the "work" of pain management for yourself.* As you create the regimen that feels most right for you—body, mind, and spirit—you will probably feel increasingly glad to have "taken the reins."

A Note about Case Examples

In the pages to follow, you will read several examples of different peo-ple's journeys with regard to pain, including their symptoms, emotional challenges and strengths, relationship struggles, communication styles, and selection of therapeutic approaches. In some cases, the examples are based on individual patients whose personal details have been changed suf-ficiently to protect their privacy. In most cases, the person featured is a com-posite of several individuals who have struggled with a common symptom, challenge, or theme. But all of the case examples are presented to reflect accurately the very relatable and real-world experiences of those striving to manage pain and all that comes with it.

Mary's Journey

Mary sought treatment with biofeedback to manage her chronic lower back pain and related anxiety. Although her physical therapist recom-mended stretching at home or taking a gentle yoga class, Mary was ini-tially resistant to these ideas as she said she could not imagine feeling well enough to do so. Yet, after doing biofeedback weekly in the office and daily at-home relaxation practice for two months, she reported feeling noticeably less pain. As a result, her doctor gave Mary clearance to decrease the dose of some of her pain medications. As Mary's pain and anxiety improved, she felt more receptive to adding gentle yoga stretches to her regimen. Later, she increased the length and frequency of her meditation practice because she noticed that this, too, helped her feel better in general.

"Meditation is one of the few things I do just for me. I feel a sense of peace when I meditate that helps me deal with everything else in my life."

Although she still experienced pain flare-ups from time to time, Mary noticed that her integrative approach felt like a gift she could give herself that had benefits beyond decreasing her pain intensity ratings and improv-ing her ability to cope with pain. Monthly visits to her pain doctor decreased to bimonthly and then quarterly, with as-needed check-ins depending on how she was feeling and the medications she was taking. Mary assumed her rightful place as the most influential member of her pain management team.

Rating Pain Severity

Each pain provider you see, both CAM and conventional, will likely assess your pain severity, frequency, and quality according to a specific scale. Reporting your pain at each visit helps your doctor assess if and how your pain changes over time, for better or worse. A commonly used scale is the zero to ten rating, with zero representing "no pain at all" and ten meaning "the worst possible pain." Another option is to rate pain severity on a three-point scale, where one equals "mild," two equals "moderate," and three equals "severe." Yet another scale in common use is the FACES pain scale, which usually ranges from zero to ten but sometimes is scaled from zero to five, and in either case features a series of cartoon faces depicting increasing pain and distress.

If you prefer a visual approach to rating your pain, yet another option is a visual analog scale, or VAS. A VAS is simply a horizontal line drawn on a piece of paper, with a zero at the left end and 100 at the right end. When presented with a VAS, you place a vertical mark through the line representing the severity of your pain, with zero representing no pain and 100 the worst pain possible. VASs are sometimes used in hospital settings or when assessing pain for a clinical study; some people prefer to use these rather than the other rating scales previously mentioned.

The Importance of "Two Points"

In general, a two-point change on a ten-point scale, or a change of 20 percent, is considered to be a "clinically significant improvement." Often, pain relief happens over time as you find and develop increasing skill using the right combination of therapies for you. Even if you hope for a large reduction in pain, know that the two-point change from a pain rating of ten down to an eight, and an eight down to a six, is meaningful and a good sign!

Pain Diaries

It's helpful, especially at the beginning of your pain journey, to keep a pain diary of some sort. A pain diary is a cognitive-behavioral tool to help you get to know the "rhythm" of your pain—its typical ebb and flow, when or why it spikes, which therapies are helpful, and which aren't. You will read more about cognitive-behavioral therapy, or CBT, in another chapter, but it's worth knowing that although technically it is considered conventional, CBT is a nonmedical therapy and an invaluable part of an integrative pain management approach. The information you will learn from keeping a pain diary not only will help you more effectively and purposefully manage your pain but also help your doctor and other providers better understand how to help you.

You can keep a pain diary in a simple notebook, create a template on your computer, or use one of the many smartphone apps available. Because your mood, thoughts, and health behaviors affect your pain, this diary prompts you to note these as well. Here is a sample template that you can copy and use to record your diary.

PAIN AND MOOD DIARY							
Date	Time	Pain Location/ Severity 0–10	Thoughts/ Feelings	Event (Trigger)	Action (What I did)	Pain Severity 0–10	Comments

There's an App for That

If you are more technologically inclined, you may prefer to use smartphone apps to track your pain. Where applicable throughout this book, you will find a listing of no- to low-cost apps to help you monitor symptoms, progress toward your goals, or track other information relevant to your pain management program. The following are apps that can be used in lieu of an "old-school" paper pain diary. They allow you to keep track of pain intensity, frequency, duration, triggers, and more.

- My Pain Diary: Chronic Pain and Symptom Tracker is a low-cost app ($5.99 as of this writing) that is available for iOS and Android. The app allows you to track your pain symptoms and triggers, remedies, patterns, and trends. It also allows you to track the weather and take photos if these are relevant. You can even create reports to note your progress or show to your providers. Visit *http://chronicpainapp.com* for information.

- Chronic Pain Tracker Lite is the free version of this app, which limits diary entries to twenty. After that, you will need to either purchase diary expansion packs or upgrade to the Pro version, which as of this writing costs $9.99. Both versions are available for iOS only. Both allow you to record key information about your pain symptoms, triggers, and the like, and also export a PDF for printing or e-mailing to your doctor. For more information, visit *http://chronicpaintracker.com*.

- WebMD Pain Coach is free and available for iOS and Android. It also offers tracking specific to several common pain conditions as well as general monitoring of pain. You can track symptoms, triggers, and treatments and access articles, videos, and information on content relevant to your specific condition. For more information, visit *www.webmd .com/mobile*.

- Pain Diary: Catch My Pain is a free app available for both iOS and Android. Like the others mentioned, this app features engaging ways to track pain and other symptoms and enables you to share your information with your providers or family members. In addition, the app lets you monitor your happiness, stress, and fatigue; track weather conditions that impact your pain; and the like. A notable feature is the ability to track your medications with barcode scanning. For more information, visit *www.catchmypain.com*.

CHAPTER 2

Conventional Medical Treatments

Even if your goal is to minimize reliance on medical treatments, it's important to know about the conventional options for managing pain, as an integrative approach is about finding the regimen that works best for you at a given time—conventional, CAM, or combined. A number of common medications and devices used to treat pain are covered in this chapter. Your medical team will be able to provide additional information about the risks and benefits associated with each, as well as let you know about conventional medical approaches not described here.

Conventional As Part of Integrative

As you have probably surmised, your primary care medical doctor and pain medicine specialist are most likely to recommend medications, physical therapy, devices, or, if these aren't sufficiently helpful, a procedure to help you manage pain. Ideally, they will have been informed by the latest research and their clinical experience, and will be able to tell you which conventional treatments are most effective and have the lowest risk of side effects for your pain condition. Your doctor may solely recommend conventional therapies or may recommend that you use them in combination with natural therapies, as long as these seem appropriate for your health issues and will not interact negatively with other treatments you are prescribed.

Medications for Pain Management

Medications are often a first line of treatment for managing chronic pain and the inflammation, mood symptoms, and sleep issues that so often accompany it. When used properly and under careful supervision, medications may make an important difference in how you feel and how able you are to do what you need to. Oftentimes, people who express an interest in integrative medicine may prefer a "natural," medication-free approach. This is a valid stance to take if your pain is managed well enough with other therapies and your mood and overall health and functioning are fairly good. You may also choose an alternative-therapies approach if you have tried conventional treatments and failed to experience adequate benefit.

When to Consider Medication

If you haven't achieved sufficient relief despite your best efforts, or find that you are not able to function reasonably well at work, at home, or socially, or if your pain continues to interfere with your ability to do the things that are most important to you, it's worth talking to your doctor about medications that could address your more stubborn and bothersome symptoms.

For all medications mentioned in the sections that follow, the generic and most common brand names (in parentheses) are provided. If a medication is only available in generic form, no brand name will be listed.

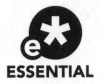

ESSENTIAL

Many people worry that they will have to take a specific drug "forever." The right medication may be what enables you to take the edge off your symptoms enough to engage in the other therapies described in this book. It's possible that this decrease in symptoms and increase in use of other pain management therapies will ultimately enable you to decrease, change, or discontinue medication.

NSAIDs and Acetaminophen

The term "NSAID" stands for "nonsteroidal anti-inflammatory drug." Often this class of medication may be the first you try, as many are available over the counter as well as by prescription. Most NSAIDs work by blocking COX-1 and COX-2 enzymes; however, some newer NSAIDs block COX-2 more selectively and COX-1 less. COX-1 and COX-2 enzymes are involved in the making of hormone-like compounds, called prostaglandins, that are implicated in both inflammation and pain. COX-1 enzymes are also involved in the production of the protective mucus in your gastrointestinal (GI) tract, so taking NSAIDs can lead to GI ulcers and bleeding.

NSAIDs are frequently taken for headaches and arthritis, among other pain conditions. Common NSAIDs include: aspirin (Bayer), ibuprofen (Motrin, Advil), and naproxen (Aleve). Examples of prescription NSAIDs are naproxen (Naprosyn), and ketorolac (Toradol). Celecoxib (Celebrex), nabumetone (Relafen), and meloxicam (Mobic) are examples of newer types of NSAIDs, referred to as selective COX-2 inhibitors.

Acetaminophen (Tylenol) is not an NSAID, but is included here because it is available over the counter and as such is often confused with NSAIDs. Acetaminophen is used to reduce pain and fever but will not reduce swelling and inflammation like NSAIDs do. Nor is it as prone to cause stomach upset. Acetaminophen is combined with both aspirin and caffeine under the brand Excedrin.

NSAIDs are generally very safe when taken for occasional pain according to the dosage listed on the package, or according to your doctor's recommendations. NSAIDs increase the risk of gastrointestinal bleeding, however, which can be dangerous and in very rare cases fatal. People who have kidney disease, problems with blood clotting or who take blood thinners, have blood pressure issues, liver, or cardiac diseases, or who have stomach ulcers should not use NSAIDs for pain. NSAIDs can also cause severe allergic reactions.

Many over-the-counter medications contain the NSAID aspirin, including BC Powder, Alka-Seltzer, and Aspergum, to name a few. Although this book is written for adults in pain, it is worth noting that aspirin should never be given to a child unless with the specific recommendation of your child's physician because of the risk of Reye's syndrome, a potentially fatal reaction.

COX-2 inhibitors are thought to be gentler to the GI tract because they don't have the same effect on COX-1; however, they are not without potential risks, including increased risk of heart attack and stroke.

The most common side effects associated with acetaminophen are rash and nausea. Acetaminophen is sometimes combined with opioid pain medications (to make Vicodin and Percocet), and with aspirin and caffeine (Excedrin), to enhance their analgesic effect. It is also found in many over-the-counter cold and flu remedies (e.g., Alka-Seltzer Plus, Robitussin, Theraflu), as well as in products for menstrual pain (e.g., Midol).

The FDA recommends that adults not exceed 4,000 mg of acetaminophen in a 24-hour period, and many doctors have recommended that the maximum daily dose be lowered to 3,250 mg. Ideally you should strive to take less if pain relief is achieved with a lower daily total, as too much acetaminophen can cause liver and kidney damage. If you are taking any other pain medications, whether over-the-counter, prescription, or both, you are at greater risk of taking too much acetaminophen. Be sure to read medication labels so you know exactly how much acetaminophen you are ingesting from all sources on any given day.

Ideally, NSAIDs and acetaminophen will be used short-term. NSAIDs can also make breathing more difficult if you have asthma or are prone to asthma attacks. Finally, do not use acetaminophen or NSAIDs if you have kidney or liver problems or consume excessive amounts of alcohol.

ALERT

According to the FDA, Americans purchased more than 28 billion doses of products containing acetaminophen in 2005 alone. The safety margin of this drug is narrow, however, and taking even a small amount over the maximum can cause liver injury, including liver failure or death. So, although it is a very commonly used over-the-counter medicine, acetaminophen needs to be taken with care.

Corticosteroid Drugs

Corticosteroids, also referred to as steroids, are used to suppress inflammation and can reduce pain. Steroids may be prescribed to treat a variety of conditions, including lupus, arthritis, asthma, allergies, muscle and disc inflammation, and inflammatory bowel conditions. Some steroids include: dexamethasone (Baycadron or Decadron), prednisone, and methylprednisolone. Steroids can be prescribed for use topically, orally, as an inhaler, and via injection. The type of delivery depends on the condition being treated.

Side effects of steroids over weeks and months may include thinning skin that bruises easily and is slow to heal, swelling, brittle bones, immune issues, weight gain, changes in blood sugar, changes to the function of your adrenal glands, mood swings, and glaucoma, among others. When used for five to seven days in a "burst" or "Medrol Dosepak," you may feel a surge of energy, an increase in appetite, and have difficulty sleeping.

ALERT

If you have a diagnosis of bipolar disorder or take lithium, remind your prescribing clinician that NSAIDs are contraindicated (when a drug may be harmful to the patient), and steroids can exacerbate symptoms of mania. Dialoging with your physician about medications prescribed by other providers is essential to keeping you well.

You should only be on steroids long term if your doctor determines that the benefits outweigh the risks for you. She may also recommend you take additional calcium and vitamin D to reduce the impact of steroids on your bones. You may be advised to alter your diet to reduce the amount of weight gained while on steroid medications. If you and your doctor determine you can reduce or discontinue using steroids, you will be advised to do so gradually, under her supervision, to avoid unpleasant side effects associated with reduced adrenal hormone production.

Opioid (Narcotic) Medications

Opioids can be naturally occurring, such as opium, which was first derived thousands of years ago from the sap of the poppy plant, to semisynthetic and synthetic opioids developed more recently. Typically, drugs in this category are prescribed to treat moderate-to-severe pain that has not responded to other medications or is not likely to respond in the future. Opioids in combination with acetaminophen may be prescribed for acute pain, such as after you have had a root canal or surgery. Opioids in combination with a steroid or NSAID may be prescribed for ongoing pain such as cancer pain, or other chronic pain that has not responded well enough to other drugs alone.

Opioid drugs work by binding to special receptors in the brain, spinal cord, and other areas of the body to reduce the sensation of pain. Genetics may influence how you will respond to this class of medication, and you may also have unique responses to different types of opioids. In addition, opioids are considered either short acting, meaning that you will feel their effects relatively quickly but they will also wear off relatively quickly (within 8 hours or less), or long acting. Examples of short-acting medications include codeine, hydrocodone (Vicodin, Lortab), hydromorphone (Dilaudid), and immediate release oxycodone (Oxecta), or oxycodone plus acetaminophen (Percocet).

FACT

Addiction is different from tolerance or dependence, and results in craving other effects of the medication (e.g., "getting high," feeling detached, feeling sedated) and using it for purposes other than pain relief. Tell your doctor if you have a history of addiction to alcohol, recreational drugs, or other prescription medications before beginning an opioid regimen.

Long-acting opioids may be prescribed for pain that is ongoing or lasts most of the day, and are often taken at twelve-hour intervals. Long-acting opioids have a slower onset than short-acting ones. Some examples of long-acting opioids include morphine (MS Contin), oxycodone extended release (OxyContin), and methadone.

Although effective for some types of pain, opioids are not considered a first line of treatment for neuropathic pain. Some people will find they develop tolerance to opioids, which means that over time they need more medication to achieve the same analgesic effect. Opioid medications also have the potential to lead to dependence, where you will experience significant withdrawal symptoms if you stop taking the drug abruptly. This is *not* the same thing as addiction.

Possible side effects associated with opioids include constipation, nausea and vomiting, itching (pruritus), feeling sedated, changes in your mood and thinking, and respiratory depression (slowed breathing). Your doctor will probably aim to reduce the risk of side effects by starting you at a low dose and increasing it slowly until you achieve sufficient pain relief. If you take an opioid medication regularly for more than five to seven days, your doctor will likely taper your regimen gradually in order to avoid withdrawal symptoms.

ALERT

Talk to your doctor about any conditions that may increase the risk of serious side effects from opioids, including sleep apnea, other respiratory problems, or kidney problems. In addition, you must avoid alcohol and use extreme caution when taking certain additional medications, such as benzodiazepines, while simultaneously taking opioids.

Antiepileptic Drugs

Antiepileptic drugs, also referred to as anticonvulsants, are considered appropriate first-line treatments for neuropathic pain such as postherpetic neuralgia, trigeminal neuralgia, diabetic peripheral neuropathy, and other types of nerve pain. They are also prescribed for functional pain syndromes such as fibromyalgia and, much less commonly, functional abdominal pain. Examples of antiepileptics used for pain are carbamazepine (Tegretol), gabapentin (Neurontin, Gralise), topiramate (Topamax), pregabalin (Lyrica), and oxcarbazepine (Trileptal).

It's not known exactly how antiepileptic medications might help with pain, but it's possible that they block pain in the brain and spinal cord and possibly in the periphery (nerves outside those in the brain and spinal cord), as well.

The American Academy of Pain Medicine acknowledges that these drugs demonstrate moderate ability at best to ease neuropathic pain. Another source of information about health related topics such as medications and some CAM therapies is Cochrane. Cochrane is a global network of researchers, professionals, patients, and others, many of who are renowned in their fields. They endeavor to review and summarize research on a variety of medical and scientific topics. They function independently of drug manufacturers and other companies, and do not accept commercial funding. Cochrane reviews are considered to be credible and understandable summaries of the science.

A 2013 Cochrane review of antiepileptic drugs found that there is some evidence that gabapentin and pregabalin were effective for long-term pain management of diabetic peripheral neuropathy and postherpetic neuralgia. Pregabalin was also found to help with post-stroke pain, other central neuropathic pain, and fibromyalgia. The review concluded that between 10 and 40 percent of people with these conditions who take gabapentin or pregabalin will achieve about a 50 percent improvement in their pain, but that most people would get no pain relief from these medications.

In addition, most people taking gabapentin or pregabalin experienced side effects, and about a quarter of the people taking these drugs had side effects that were so difficult to tolerate that they stopped taking the drugs. Yet, serious side effects were no more common in people taking gabapentin or pregabalin than in those taking a placebo (a "sugar pill"). The Cochrane review also concluded that there was a lack of evidence that antiepileptic drugs were helpful for neuropathic pain and fibromyalgia.

These findings mean that there is some evidence that antiepileptic drugs will help a small to medium subset of people with neuropathic or functional pain to some extent. Most people who are prescribed antiepileptic drugs for pain are likely to discontinue taking them due to unpleasant side effects. That said, some people will experience sufficient benefits that warrant taking these medications.

Despite the Cochrane conclusion, the American Academy of Pain Medicine states that carbamazepine has been shown in clinical trials to provide significant relief, at least initially, to up to 80 percent of those who have trigeminal neuralgia. This effect may not be lasting, however.

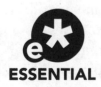

ESSENTIAL

In 2008, the FDA concluded that taking an antiepileptic was associated with an increased risk of suicidal thoughts or behavior for just under 0.5 percent of patients. That is equivalent to one additional suicidal person for every 530 people treated with this type of medication. Having chronic pain itself is linked to higher rates of depression and suicidal thoughts or behavior. Talk to your doctor about whether the benefits of antiepileptics outweigh the risks.

Potential side effects of the previously mentioned antiepileptics named include headache, rashes, nausea, vomiting, swelling, changes in weight, and confusion. The FDA has also issued a warning that antiepileptics may increase the risk of suicidal thoughts and suicide. If you stop taking an anticonvulsant abruptly, you can experience withdrawal symptoms such as nausea, pain, sweating, anxiety, and insomnia, so your doctor will recommend a gradual taper if you need or decide to discontinue this medication.

Antidepressants

Although antidepressants will be discussed further in the chapter on mood and pain, this section provides an overview of the antidepressant medications prescribed for pain that show evidence of benefit for both pain and mood. The medications mentioned in this section fall into the following categories: tricyclics, selective serotonin reuptake inhibitors (SSRIs), serotonin-norepinephrine reuptake inhibitors (SNRIs), and atypical antidepressants. Antidepressants are generally well tolerated by those who take them, although there are potential side effects. Antidepressants can be used alone or in combination with other pain medications, and can be used for pain even in the absence of a mood issue. With many of these medications, the dose required for pain management is lower than that needed to achieve an antidepressant effect.

Tricyclics

Tricyclics are an older class of drugs that are considered particularly effective as compared to SSRIs and SNRIs for improving sleep continuity, deep sleep, and reduction in pain severity. They are sometimes combined with other antidepressants or other types of pain medications. Examples of tricyclics include amitriptyline, nortriptyline (Pamelor), clomipramine (Anafranil), doxepin (Sinequan), imipramine (Tofranil), and desipramine (Norpramin). Possible side effects include dry mouth, dizziness, blurred vision, sedation, constipation, tachycardia (rapid heart rate), and orthostatic hypotension (low blood pressure that happens when you stand up after having been sitting).

SSRIs and SNRIs

SSRIs and SNRIs are newer classes of antidepressants than tricyclics. Although tricyclics are considered more effective for neuropathic pain than newer drugs (which is why they are more commonly prescribed for this purpose), SSRIs and SNRIs tend to have fewer side effects. Examples of SSRIs are paroxetine (Paxil), fluoxetine (Prozac), citalopram (Celexa), and sertraline (Zoloft). Side effects of SSRIs include nausea, sleep disturbances, sexual dysfunction, headache, dry mouth, and changes in appetite. Examples of SNRIs include venlafaxine (Effexor), duloxetine (Cymbalta), and milnacipran (Savella). Potential side effects include the same side effects as listed for SSRIs, plus tachycardia and hypertension.

Atypicals

Atypical antidepressants do not fall into any of the other categories, and affect the neurotransmitters serotonin, norepinephrine, and dopamine. They include buproprion (Wellbutrin), mirtazapine (Remeron), and trazodone (Oleptro). Buproprion has been shown to be effective for neuropathic pain and can also help with smoking cessation by reducing the experience of cravings. When prescribed for this purpose, it is sold under the brand name Zyban. Like other antidepressant medications, some of these help with sleep; some may also help with anxiety. Unlike medications in other antidepressant classes, atypicals are less likely to cause sexual side effects. Some atypicals can cause loss of appetite and others, increased appetite. Your doctor can help you decide on the medication most likely to help you with the least likelihood of undesirable side effects.

FACT

Approximately 80 percent of chronic pain patients are thought to have significant problems sleeping. Disruptions in deep sleep (also called "slow-wave sleep") have been shown to increase pain sensitivity in several studies. Ongoing insomnia also is linked to persistent symptoms of depression. Because tricyclics improve slow-wave sleep better than some other medications, your doctor may prescribe this medication for sleep, pain, or both—even if you are not depressed.

Benzodiazepines

Benzodiazepines or "tranquilizers" are thought to work by increasing the amount or availability of GABA, a neurotransmitter that is associated with feeling calm. Over the past decade or more, the use of benzodiazepines in chronic pain patients has increased significantly.

Technically, medications in this class are not prescribed for pain per se, but patients who have chronic pain may often find themselves prescribed "benzos" if they report anxiety or difficulty sleeping. Specifically, your doctor may prescribe diazepam (Valium), clonazepam (Klonopin), alprazolam (Xanax), lorazepam (Ativan), or another benzodiazepine to address the following: anticipatory anxiety (worry you will have a pain spike), muscle spasms that have not responded sufficiently to prescription muscle relaxants, feelings of general distress or anxiety, and when prescription sleep medications have failed to adequately remedy insomnia.

Benzodiazepines should be used with caution, especially if you are also taking opioid pain medications. Inappropriately combining the two medications can lead to significant adverse effects or death. Similarly, you should not drink alcohol when taking medications in this class.

"Benzos" (and opioids) can make people feel a pleasant sort of detachment, which may seem especially appealing if you have been having trouble coping, but they also have the potential to cause psychological and physical dependence. If you decide to decrease the dose or discontinue benzodiazepine medications, you must decrease gradually and systematically, under a doctor's supervision, to avoid the risk of withdrawal symptoms such as seizures.

Benzodiazepines prescribed at an appropriate dose are typically safe and effective, but for the most part are not usually indicated for long-term use. If your anxiety is ongoing or very frequent, antidepressant medications are typically considered a more appropriate choice and will not leave you with the floaty, disconnected feeling you may have from benzodiazepines.

Muscle Relaxants

Just as the name implies, muscle relaxants are used to help the skeletal muscles relax. They are not a single class of medications, but rather individual drugs that each work on the central nervous system rather than directly on the muscles. Often they are prescribed for short-term use to address back pain at the beginning of physical therapy. Some muscle relaxants include carisoprodol (Soma), cyclobenzaprine (Flexeril), metaxalone (Skelaxin), baclofen, tizanidine (Zanaflex), and methocarbamol (Robaxin). The benzodiazepine diazepam (Valium) is also prescribed to treat muscle spasms.

Muscle relaxants are typically prescribed for use in the short term. They should not be combined with alcohol. Some more common side effects reported for muscle relaxants include dizziness, drowsiness, headache, irritability, nausea, nervousness, upset stomach, vomiting, or vision problems.

Carisoprodol can become habit forming. Cyclobenzaprine may cause urinary retention in males who have enlarged prostates, and can also impair mental or physical functioning. Diazepam can affect sleep cycles and also worsen depression. Baclofen can cause withdrawal symptoms, including seizures, if you discontinue abruptly after using for a long time. It can also increase your risk of developing an ovarian cyst. Tell your doctor if you have any history of kidney or liver problems before taking metaxalone or methocarbamol.

Procedures to Address Pain

When pain is severe, persistent, or extremely bothersome and has not responded to other approaches, your doctor may recommend more invasive therapies. The following sections give general information about some of the most prominent procedures used to treat pain.

Diagnostic or Therapeutic Nerve Block

A diagnostic or therapeutic nerve block is one procedure that can help determine the source of pain and also provide some relief. Nerve blocks involve infusing local anesthetics and other agents in the epidural space (an area between your spinal cord and the vertebral wall of your spine) or next to the perineural sheath (the thin protective coating around peripheral nerves). Either may provide pain relief for days to weeks, and can help specifically with pain in the spine, joints, chest, limbs, or bursae (fibrous sacs between certain tendons and nearby bones).

Nerve blocks are considered generally safe. The epidural space is vulnerable to developing epidural abscesses, however. These are infections that can impair feeling and movement if not identified and treated quickly.

Trigger Point Injections

Trigger point injections are very common procedures for certain kinds of pain. These involve injecting an anesthetic or saline, and sometimes a corticosteroid, into trigger points. Trigger points are painful knots in the muscle and fascia that can be felt with the hand. If you have an allergy to any of these medications, your doctor may use a dry-needling technique to break up the knots without using medication.

Trigger point injections can be performed quickly, are considered effective, and are low risk overall. You may experience post-injection pain, particularly if no anesthetic is injected into the trigger point, but this should resolve within a few days.

Facet Joint Blocks

Facet joint blocks, similar to trigger point injections, involve injecting anesthetic, steroids, or both into the facet joints along the spine. The anesthetic provides immediate, short-term pain relief, and the steroid addresses inflammation, possibly providing longer-term relief.

Facet joint injections are considered to have a low risk of complications. Possible ones include risk of allergic reaction to the anesthetic, bleeding, infection, soreness at the injection site, and in rare cases, nerve damage.

Neurolysis

Neurolysis involves the partial or complete destruction of nerves that are causing pain. This can be done via the injection of chemicals (e.g., alcohol, phenol, glycerol), by cryotherapy (intense cold), or radiotherapy (via intense heat). Neurolysis is used to treat neuropathic pain, as well as visceral pain due to cancer. In general, neurolysis is considered after other approaches have been tried and found ineffective.

Neurolysis is typically only performed for intractable pain, such as in the cancer setting, because the risks of complications are higher than with other therapies (including infection, numbness, paralysis, and pruritus) and because there is a high rate of pain recurrence.

Devices to Help Manage Pain

In addition to drugs and procedures, there are devices on the market that are used to help "turn down the volume" on pain. These devices generate electrical signals that, in essence, compete with pain for attention.

Transcutaneous Electrical Nerve Stimulation (TENS)

Transcutaneous electrical nerve stimulation (TENS) treats pain with the use of a small, handheld device that delivers a low-voltage electrical current to your skin via two electrodes. TENS is thought to work by sending a signal to your brain via nerve fibers associated with nonpainful touch, thereby blocking or reducing the pain signals sent from the pain-related nerve fibers in the area being treated. Another hypothesis is that TENS works by stimulating the release of endorphins—your body's natural pain-reducing chemicals. TENS is typically used to manage back or neck pain, pain in tendons or bursae, fibromyalgia, and other types of pain.

TENS is generally considered safe; however, people who have pacemakers or defibrillators should not use it. There is a small risk of the electrical current feeling too intense or causing a burn. The currents on TENS units are adjustable; your healthcare provider (frequently a physical therapist) will help you determine the appropriate setting.

Cefaly

Cefaly is a device that was developed in Canada and is designed to treat and prevent migraines. It's a type of TENS that is shaped like a headband and requires placement of an adhesive electrode on the forehead that connects to the device. Cefaly generates tiny electrical impulses to stimulate the nerve endings of the trigeminal nerve, which is thought to induce relaxation. The FDA reviewed the data on the device and subsequently allowed for its marketing in the United States in 2014.

Cefaly may cause the user to feel a tingling or massaging sensation where the electrode is applied. Cefaly is indicated for patients eighteen years of age and older and should only be used once per day for twenty minutes. The FDA's approval was in part based on data from a Belgian study of sixty-seven migraine sufferers who experienced significantly fewer days with migraines per month and used less migraine medication than those who used a placebo device. The device did not completely prevent migraines in this sample, however, and did not reduce the intensity of migraines that did occur.

When the Device Is Implanted

Implantable devices are usually tried only after other therapies have failed to produce adequate relief.

Spinal Cord Stimulation (SCS) and Peripheral Nerve Stimulation (PNS)

Spinal cord stimulation (SCS) and peripheral nerve stimulation (PNS) involve the surgical implantation of a device that provides electrical stimulation to either the spinal cord or peripheral nerves. The electrical stimulation targets the nerve fibers associated with nonpainful sensations, and is thought to inhibit the signals sent by pain fibers. During an outpatient procedure, patients receive a sedative before the doctor implants the stimulator under the skin, and then implants the wires via a needle inserted either near the spinal cord or the affected peripheral nerves. SCS and PNS are considered to be useful for chronic neuropathic pain, complex regional pain syndrome, and peripheral vascular disease.

Your doctor will do a trial of SCS or PNS using a temporary electrode and an external stimulator to make sure this treatment is helpful to you before finalizing the procedure. The stimulator may need to be reprogrammed at some point to maintain adequate coverage of the painful area. The implantation of wires and a battery pack along the spine can inhibit movement to some degree.

Risks related to SCS include the potential for scar tissue to develop, decreased effectiveness over time as your body becomes used to the stimulation, pain possibly moving beyond the area affected by the device, hardware failure, and infection.

The Stimwave Spinal Cord Stimulator

The Stimwave Freedom Spinal Cord Stimulator was approved by the Food and Drug Administration in late 2014. Like the traditional SCS, it relies on neurostimulation to reduce pain. The Stimwave is tiny in comparison, however. It is injected via needle under the skin. The Stimwave is also wireless, and with proper preparation, a person who has had a Stimwave implanted can undergo magnetic resonance imaging (MRI) if necessary. In addition, Bluetooth technology allows your doctor to program the device remotely.

Unlike the SCS, which is fully implanted, the Stimwave requires you to wear an external transmitter to power the device. Because the Stimwave has only recently been cleared for use, it will be some time before enough people have had the implant in for a sufficient period of time to definitively show how effective and safe it is in the long run.

Medication Pumps

Medication pumps, otherwise known as intrathecal drug delivery systems, allow for the delivery of medication (often opioids or medications indicated for nerve pain) to the fluid around the spinal cord via a small catheter. The pump is implanted in the abdominal wall.

Intrathecal pumps can provide pain relief when other approaches may not have, and because the medication is delivered directly to the spinal fluid, much lower doses can be used than if taken orally. Potential risks include infection, headache, the pump moving around, the equipment failing and resulting in accidental over- or under-dosing of medication, and developing a tolerance to the medications. In the event of the latter, the dose can be increased up to a certain limit. Medication pumps are usually only used in cases where pain is severe and after other methods have failed.

For more information about medical therapies for chronic pain, both those mentioned in this section as well as others, you may wish to visit the American Chronic Pain Association's website: *www.theacpa.org/Consumer-Guide*. They provide support, information, and education to chronic pain patients, family members, and healthcare professionals.

CHAPTER 3

The Physiology of Pain

As you are probably aware, the way you experience pain is the result of an interaction among your peripheral nerves, brain, and spinal cord, as well as your emotional state and how well you are coping. The complex nature of pain can make it feel challenging to treat; however, understanding how your brain and body contribute to pain and analgesia (pain relief) can put you in a better position to manage your pain and achieve better functioning.

Key Terms Related to Pain

As you read more about your chronic pain condition, and as you meet with your medical team, you will hear a number of terms related to pain that are not commonly used outside a pain management medical setting. Please feel free to refer to the following definitions as you encounter these terms:

- **Analgesia:** Relief from pain.
- **Hyperalgesia:** Increased pain from a stimulus that would normally be painful. Example: a pinprick causing extreme, intolerable pain.
- **Allodynia:** Pain caused by a stimulus that normally would not be painful at all. Example: the sensation of clothing against your skin feeling excruciating.
- **Functional Pain:** Pain that is not due to a structural problem or disease, and is not detected by normal clinical examination. Example: functional abdominal pain, irritable bowel syndrome, fibromyalgia.
- **Nociceptive Pain:** Caused by damage to tissue. Often described as throbbing, aching, dull or sharp, etc. Example: postoperative pain, pain from stubbing your toe, or a cut on the skin.
- **Somatic Pain:** Pain in the skin or tissues such as muscles and joints. Somatic pain is a type of nociceptive pain. Example: a paper cut on your skin, or a muscle strain.
- **Visceral Pain:** Pain occurring in the viscera, or organs within the body. Visceral pain is a type of nociceptive pain. Example: cancer pain or pain from a kidney stone.
- **Neuropathic Pain:** Pain resulting from damage to the peripheral nerves, such as following a serious burn, or after developing shingles. Neuropathic pain syndromes tend to produce pain that is described as painful numbness, burning, tingling, or an electrical sensation. Example: postherpetic neuralgia, diabetic peripheral neuropathy.
- **Central Pain (Central Sensitization):** Pain resulting from maladaptive changes in the brain, spinal cord, or both, rather than caused by damage to peripheral nerves. Central pain syndromes are a subtype of neuropathic pain. Complex regional pain syndrome and phantom limb pain are types of central pain syndromes.

- **Catastrophize:** To react to something extremely negatively or believe it to be worse than it actually is (i.e., to make something into a catastrophe). An example of catastrophizing is to think, "This pain is so bad; I will never be able to have a life again!" Catastrophizing is linked to increased pain severity and poorer functioning.
- **Central Nervous System (CNS):** Collectively referring to the brain, brain stem, and spinal cord.
- **Peripheral Nervous System (PNS):** The part of the nervous system that is outside the CNS, such as the nerves in the body, cranial (skull) nerves, spinal nerves, and autonomic nervous system.
- **Periphery:** Referring to the areas outside the brain, brainstem, and spinal cord, such as your limbs; areas sending signals via the PNS.
- **Viscera:** Your internal organs.
- **Autonomic Nervous System (ANS):** The nerves that "innervate" or activate the smooth and cardiac muscles and glands. Also governs actions considered involuntary, such as secretions and the functions of internal organs, as well as the movement of food through your digestive system.

Before long, these terms will become second nature to your understanding of and discussions with your team about pain.

How Pain Happens

With acute pain, nerve fibers called nociceptors communicate information up the spinal cord to the brain, where it is recognized as pain. Nociceptors are specialized sensory nerves in the periphery that are found in the skin, bones, muscles, joints, and internal organs.

One type of nociceptor, the A-delta nerve fiber, communicates the first, or "fast" pain, such as that immediate, highly unpleasant, and jarring sensation caused by stubbing your toe or bumping your "funny bone" (which clearly isn't funny in the least). Another type of nociceptor, the C fiber, is responsible for the slow, or "second," pain. Think of this as the dull, sore, more diffuse pain that comes second and lingers for a while after an injury.

FACT

Redheads have greater sensitivity to pain. The medication lidocaine is also less effective in redheads. Mutations in the melanocortin-1 receptor gene are the cause for both red hair and increased pain sensitivity. Redheads can require up to 20 percent more anesthesia than other people!

Although you probably notice the sensation of pain in the peripheral nervous system (PNS), pain is an experience that requires the brain for you to perceive it as pain at all. And that is both bad and good news. The "bad" part is that there is considerable overlap across a number of areas of the brain that interpret pain and also are involved with memory, emotion, and the meaning you attribute to pain. Consequently, your emotional state and thoughts about pain can increase the perceived severity of pain and also leave you feeling like you cannot cope with the pain you have.

The "good news" is that your brain is a very powerful tool for changing the pain experience. In fact, your brain can be your strongest ally in helping turn down the intensity of your pain, enhance your ability to cope with the situation you find yourself in, and make good decisions about how to manage your pain.

The Brain Controls the Pain

In short, your brain is what tells you that you are experiencing pain at all. Your brain also decides whether or not the pain is something you feel you can manage. The brain looks for ways to make sense of the pain experience via memories and your emotional response to pain, and decides how (and whether) to move forward or not despite being in pain. In addition, as mentioned previously, your brain can experience pain *even despite a lack of damage* to tissue anywhere in the body.

Sometimes a pain disorder results from damage to or dysfunction of the central nervous system (CNS). This dysfunction can be caused by a stroke, tumor, epilepsy, Parkinson's disease, limb amputation, or multiple sclerosis. Damage to the CNS can cause you to feel constant, moderate to severe pain that is often characterized as burning or tingling, with painful numbness. The pain can be localized to a small area such as your face or a hand, but can also affect a larger area of your body. When your pain is attributable to central nervous system changes, it is considered a central pain syndrome (CPS).

FACT

About 5–10 percent of people who have a limb amputated wind up seeking treatment for phantom limb pain, although some sources estimate that phantom limb pain occurs in as many as 80 percent or more of people who lose a body part.

Pain disorders that fall into the category of CPS can be especially challenging to tolerate. One reason is that even things that would normally not cause pain, such as gentle touch, can feel excruciating. Medications alone are typically only partly effective for managing CPSs. The most effective treatments for most CPSs include a combination of specific medications such as antidepressants and anticonvulsants, mind-body approaches, and sometimes physical therapy.

Exorcising the "Ghost" of Phantom Limb Pain

The issue of phantom limb pain provides useful examples of both how CNS changes can cause very real pain in another area and how you can achieve relief via your mind and brain. Even if you do not have phantom limb pain, or pain in a limb that has been amputated, it's worth knowing how a deceptively simple mind-body treatment has helped sufferers achieve relief where conventional treatments have been largely ineffective.

Although the term "limb" is used, phantom limb pain can occur after the loss of other parts as well, including an eye, tongue, bladder, penis, and more. Not to be confused with pain in the remaining tissue at the site of amputation, phantom limb pain is experienced as cramping, aching, burning, or electrical shock sensations in the part that has been removed.

This condition causes significant distress in the sufferer and, like other types of pain, is worsened by stress or mood issues.

Doctors originally assumed that phantom limb pain was purely psychological in origin; however, it is now known that very real changes in the spinal cord and brain fool the mind into thinking that the missing part is both present and in significant pain. The resulting experience of pain is quite real!

Risks for developing phantom limb pain include older age and pain in the limb prior to amputation. Mind-body approaches such as hypnosis, biofeedback, and imagery have shown some success in treating phantom limb pain. One of the newest mind-body treatments, however, is something called "mirror box therapy." Developed by Dr. V.S. Ramachandran, this treatment uses a simple and inexpensive box-and-mirror combination that allows the patient's brain to "see" the missing limb and "unclench" a tight fist, "flex" a cramped foot, and the like. This happens via the mirror's reflecting the image of the intact limb in such a way that it appears that the missing limb is still present.

Mirror Neurons and Mirror Box Therapy

Mirror box therapy is thought to work at least in part due to the activation of "mirror neurons" in the brain. A mirror neuron is a special type of brain cell that is active when you observe another person engaging in an activity. In fact, if you watch someone else ride a bike, the motor and other relevant areas of your brain will become more active, almost as if *you* are the one riding. Similarly, if you consider the example of someone who has lost their left leg and is now experiencing pain, placing that person's right leg in the mirror box allows his brain to visualize and experience the missing left leg as though it is still present. Patients have reported feeling emotional and physical relief from moving or massaging the intact limb, and feeling very clearly that they are doing so with the missing part.

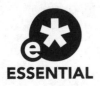
Recently, doctors at Veterans Affairs medical centers have begun using mirror box therapy for veterans who report phantom limb pain and have not responded well to other treatments. You can watch a news clip of a veteran undergoing successful treatment with mirror box therapy by visiting this link: *www.youtube.com/watch?v=YL_6OMPywnQ.*

Gate Control Theory of Pain

In the 1960s, two scientists, Patrick Wall and Ronald Melzack, developed what is known as the Gate Control Theory of Pain. Without going into too much technical detail, a simple way of understanding the Gate Control Theory is that signals sent via pain-transmitting (nociceptor) and non-pain-transmitting (A-beta) nerve fibers essentially must pass through a theoretical "gate" in the dorsal horn, or rear, of the spinal cord to reach the brain. If the strength of the signals from the nociceptors is greater than that of those sent via other nerve fibers, they will make it through the gate, their information will be communicated to various structures in the brain, and you will feel pain. If the information sent by non-pain-related nerve fibers is more prominent, however, and gets through the gate first, this will block some or all of the pain sensation.

Opening and Closing the Gate

You will probably hear your pain providers talking about things that open and close the gate. Factors thought to open the gate and make way for pain include:

- Prolonged inactivity
- Poor pacing of activities (e.g., overdoing it)
- Injury
- Long-term narcotic use
- Poor posture
- Anxiety
- Depression
- Catastrophizing
- General stress
- Loneliness

Things that close the gate and can reduce pain include:

- Distraction
- Positive mood
- Good stress management
- The right type(s) and dose of medication
- Mind-body techniques such as mindfulness and other types of meditation, hypnosis, and other types of relaxation training
- Stimulation of non-pain nerves in the periphery such as via TENS or massage

Mind-body practices in particular send a competing signal from your brain to the body, and change the interpretation and even block some of the pain signal being relayed from the spinal cord up to the brain. Thus, mind-body practices are types of "top down" techniques.

FACT

A six-year study of mindfulness-based stress reduction with chronic pain patients found that mindfulness was linked to significantly reduced pain, better functioning, and a decrease in psychological distress. Other studies have found mindfulness to reduce pain severity by over 50 percent! And in general, mindfulness enhances calm and focus.

It's worth noting that the type of relaxation achieved through practices like mindfulness and other types of meditation, hypnosis, and biofeedback is different from simply "relaxing." Watching TV or reading a book can provide a welcome distraction (as can mind-body practices), and may also reduce your pain or make it feel more tolerable by taking your mind off it. But the overall effect is different from the profound peace and comfort that can be cultivated by the mind-body practices mentioned and also described in further detail later in this book.

The Race Through the Gate

A way that may help you visualize the Gate Control Theory is to think of a narrow waterway with lots of different boats racing to a drawbridge (the pain gate). Beyond the drawbridge is the finish line (the brain), and whichever boat gets there first will limit or block the others' access.

If the boats in a particular race are the *SS Back Pain*, the *TENS*, and the partying *Day(boat) of Our Lives*, the *SS Back Pain* may start out in the lead, but the *TENS* and *Day(boat)* may steadily gain on it, racing valiantly to try to beat *Back Pain* to the brain. If either the *TENS* or the *Day(Boat)* makes it through the drawbridge first, *Back Pain* won't win, and might not even make it through at all.

In a "top down" scenario, the *SS Back Pain* may be racing up the waterway trying to reach the brain, but be headed off by the graceful sailboat

Hypno-Therapy, sailing down from the brain and lowering the drawbridge, thus closing the pain gate and blocking *Back Pain*'s access.

The Gate Control Theory is not a perfect one, but it can be helpful in understanding why, when you stub your toe, your instinct is to grab and rub it, as well as why mind-body therapies can blunt or block pain signals.

Factors That Increase Your Risk of Chronic Pain

Over the past several decades, much research has been conducted on the factors associated with the development of chronic pain, as well as those associated with increasing pain severity by opening the pain gate. Although there is much that is still not well understood about pain, some of these factors are as follows:

- Underweight (BMI <18.5)
- Overweight (BMI >25.0)
- Smoking
- Anxiety
- Depression
- Hormonal fluctuations
- Genetic factors
- Vitamin D deficiency
- Being female

In addition to this list, a number of pain syndromes tend to co-occur, meaning that if you have one, you are more likely to also have others. Examples of pain disorders and other health problems that tend to co-occur include irritable bowel syndrome (IBS), chronic widespread pain, chronic fatigue syndrome (CFS), fibromyalgia, dry eye disease, and pelvic pain.

FACT

In February 2015, the Institute of Medicine coined a new name for CFS: "systemic exertion intolerance disease." Researchers found that people who have CFS show abnormal changes in the gray and white matter and widespread inflammation in specific areas of their brains. These findings may someday shed light on the origins or nature of this illness.

The Role of Inflammation in Pain and Depression

Inflammation plays a role in many painful conditions, including arthritis, lupus, and other autoimmune disorders, as well as GI issues, skin problems, allergies, diabetes, cardiovascular disease, and cancer. When you are injured or ill, proteins called cytokines increase inflammation in your body. A certain amount of inflammation can help your body heal, but too much for too long can be problematic.

Rates of depression are higher in people who have an inflammatory illness, and an emerging line of research has also found an association between inflammation and depression and, in particular, with depression that is more severe or harder to treat. Since depression is linked to elevated inflammation, you may be wondering if taking an NSAID would also help depression symptoms. Dr. Andrew Miller of Emory University was curious about this as well. He and his colleagues found that adding an anti-inflammatory medication to an antidepressant was only helpful for those patients who were both depressed *and* had higher levels of inflammation, however. Combining an anti-inflammatory drug with an antidepressant actually made those who were depressed but had normal levels of inflammation *less* likely to respond to the antidepressant. Therefore, it is not recommended to add an NSAID to your antidepressant regimen without your doctor assessing your levels of inflammatory markers.

"Alleviators" and "Aggravators" of Chronic Pain

A basic cornerstone of pain management is assessing two key elements: what makes your pain worse (i.e., aggravators) and what makes it better (alleviators). Having a clearer understanding of what impacts your pain can give you greater control over your pain. In essence, the information in this book about what pain is, how it works, and which integrative therapies can be helpful is about alleviating and aggravating factors.

You may already be aware of what tends to worsen your pain and what usually helps you to either feel decreased pain severity or improved ability to cope. Although these factors can vary depending on the pain condition you have and because of individual differences, some common ones are listed as follows. You may wish to refer back to these lists when you begin charting your personal alleviators and aggravators:

COMMON PAIN AGGRAVATORS

- Too little sleep/fatigue
- Under-eating
- Too much caffeine
- Catastrophizing
- Depression, anxiety, distress
- Hormonal fluctuations
- Medication overuse
- Muscle tightness
- Movement/overexertion
- Being too sedentary
- Smoking

Gender Differences in Pain

Women are much more likely to seek treatment for chronic pain than men are, and also tend to report greater pain intensity. There are several reasons for this, as well as a great deal that is not known about why women are more likely to be diagnosed with chronic pain. One reason is that certain pain conditions—such as menstrual pain, vulvodynia, and endometriosis—only affect women. Yet, several conditions that affect both men and women, such as fibromyalgia, migraines, interstitial cystitis, temperomandibular joint disorder, and knee pain, occur much more often in women.

Even though women are much more likely to be diagnosed with most of the pain disorders that affect both sexes, men have been disproportionately more likely to be research study participants (this has even been true when using mice in pain research!). Including more female participants in pain studies could lead to more specialized ways of treating pain.

What Accounts for the Gender Difference?

One possible explanation is that some combination of biological factors predispose women to greater risk of developing a pain condition, poorer response to pain medications, or changes in the way pain is transmitted from the nerves to the brain. Another is that women may have a biologically-based heightened sensitivity to pain (i.e., a lower tolerance), although data are conflicting about this hypothesis.

Another possibility is that depression and anxiety make women more vulnerable to pain. This hypothesis comes from the data showing that women are more likely to be diagnosed with anxiety or depression, and both of these states increase pain severity and decrease pain coping.

Finally, it is possible that social rather than biological differences are responsible. Specifically, women are more likely to take on multiple roles, including employment, managing a home, and caring for children and aging family members. These demands place increased emotional and physical strain on women and leave far less time for self-care. In addition, if men are socialized to be stoic and strong, this may lead them to minimize pain when reporting it to others, and decrease the likelihood of seeking treatment.

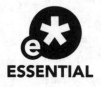

ESSENTIAL

It's unclear whether female hormones play a role in pain sensitivity. Although women seem to have a higher pain tolerance during the first half of the menstrual cycle, and it's been suggested that estrogen and progesterone decrease pain sensitivity, neither has been proven definitively.

The bottom line is that, regardless of gender, practicing self-care in the forms of a healthy diet, adequate sleep, exercise appropriate for your condition, and a regular stress management practice (such as meditation) can help you cope with the challenges of having both pain *and* the stresses of daily life.

If you are female, it's worth keeping a journal to see if you experience changes in pain severity, duration, or coping during the different phases of your menstrual cycle. If you are postmenopausal, note whether and how hormone replacement therapy impacts your pain. Also, be aware that your doctor may need to adjust the dose or type of pain medication you take to optimize your response to treatment.

Finally, practice effective communication with family members and others with regard to sharing of household chores, childcare, and the like to help decrease feelings of frustration, stress, and fatigue.

CHAPTER 4

Emotional and Social Aspects of Pain

Pain is a whole-person, whole-life experience and impacts multiple areas of your life, including your mood, self-esteem, and relationships. And as the number of painful conditions you have increases, or the longer you are in pain, the more likely it is that you will also notice feeling sad, anxious, or hopeless about the changes pain has made in your life. These feelings are totally understandable and quite common, but remember, you *can* do a lot to work with the social and emotional challenges brought on by pain.

Pain and Mood

You may already have sensed that rates of depression and anxiety are higher in those who have chronic pain than in the general population. Feeling down can make functioning in general much more difficult. If your emotions are overwhelming, they can exacerbate sensations of pain and decrease the likelihood that you will do things to help you feel better, such as exercising, eating well, taking prescribed medications, practicing relaxation, using CAM therapies, and engaging in meaningful social activities.

Depression

Depression is a topic many people shy away from talking about, but it's especially important to talk about depression symptoms for a number of reasons. In addition to depression's impact on your ability to function day to day, depression is associated with increased health risks, particularly if you also happen to have a cardiovascular illness. For example, if you have had a heart attack, you are much more likely to have an additional heart attack and other heart-related health problems. If you are depressed, you are more likely to die within the year after your heart attack. Although researchers aren't entirely sure why this is the case, one important reason may be that both depression and heart disease are related to inflammation. And as mentioned previously, depression is one factor that opens the pain gate.

Sometimes, when someone has experienced low mood for quite a while, they will fail to recognize the difference between what thoughts, feelings, and facts are "true" and which have become distorted through the lens of depression. In effect, people can "get used to" feeling down to the point that they can't remember ever having felt or thought any different. In fact, it is well known among mental health professionals that depressed people tend to have a memory bias when recalling previous events. In essence, they are more likely to remember negative events and feelings even when asked to recall positive or emotionally neutral information.

The "Hamster Wheel" of Rumination

If you are or have been depressed previously, you may also have noticed having the tendency to ruminate, or remain compulsively focused on what is difficult, disappointing, or painful. The problem with rumination is that it sets up a kind of vicious cycle of feeling bad, reflecting on things that have gone wrong, feeling even worse, and so forth.

In effect, rumination can make you feel like the Bill Murray character in the 1993 movie *Groundhog Day*. Essentially, every morning he woke up to another version of the same day, unable to figure out how to move forward in time. When you feel down in the dumps it may seem pointless to do things that you might otherwise understand would help you feel better, such as getting on a regular sleep schedule, engaging in hobbies you used to enjoy, moving your body, and getting together with friends. And the more entrenched unhealthy habits become, the more challenging it will feel to change them.

The following list will help you determine if you are experiencing symptoms of depression:

HOW TO RECOGNIZE DEPRESSION
- Difficulty concentrating or making decisions
- Changes in appetite or eating
- Fatigue and decreased energy
- Loss of interest in activities you once enjoyed
- Problems sleeping—getting either too much or too little
- Irritability
- Feelings of guilt or worthlessness
- Persistent sadness
- Feelings of wanting to die—either passively, such as not wanting to wake up, or actively, such as thinking about harming or killing yourself

ALERT

People who have a chronic pain condition are two to five times more likely to suffer from depression than people in the general population. This ranges from about 35 percent of those with pain who are seen in mental health clinics to 78 percent seen in dental clinic settings. Yet depression is often unaddressed or untreated, leading to worse pain and functioning.

Help-Rejecting Complaining

Help-rejecting complaining is the psychological term for repeatedly asking others for help, but then systematically rejecting all suggestions offered. Many people do this routinely, without realizing they are doing so. Unfortunately, friends and family who may genuinely want to help will usually wind up feeling frustrated, hopeless, and ineffectual—perhaps many of the things that the help-rejecting complainer (or HRC) is feeling, whether consciously or unconsciously.

The reason behind help-rejecting may be that the HRC is unaware of two competing parts of himself—the part that really wants things to get better and the part that either believes positive change is impossible or feels undeserving of good things. Another barrier to change may be that the HRC believes on some level that his feelings of distress will be invalidated in some way if his problem turns out to be solvable. Specifically, the HRC may fear that if change truly is possible, this will make it seem to others that his problem was somehow less "real," severe, or overwhelming than it has felt to him.

Yet another possible barrier to making change can come from the HRC believing on some level that accepting help and making change based on another's suggestions will make him feel foolish or inadequate for not having done so sooner. In other cases, the HRC may have become identified with his problems and the (sort of) "special" status that can come with having the most difficult situation of anyone around.

Even though the HRC certainly suffers, there can be many things working below the level of conscious awareness that get in the way of his being able to make good use of the help he seeks.

Phil's Crystal Ball

Phil sought treatment for his ongoing recurrent neck pain and sciatic pain that didn't respond sufficiently to medications or injections. It soon became clear to his therapist, however, that Phil's primary "pain in the neck" was his relationship with his wife of thirty-five years. Phil constantly spoke about how his wife was not affectionate with him, didn't make enough time for him, and wasn't sympathetic enough to his pain. He catastrophized frequently: "*I am just never going to be happy* unless she realizes I need to feel more important to her!" He also very frequently and with great conviction predicted, "I am never going to get better. I just *know* it. It's like I have a crystal ball that shows me the future, and it's not going to change."

Among the recommendations Phil received were to voice his feelings to his wife in a loving, nonjudgmental way ("She won't pay attention unless I'm brutally honest with her."), to invite his wife to join him in a therapy session ("No, she'll never do that. She has tennis on Wednesdays, anyway."), to write her a letter so he could share his feelings constructively and without getting angry ("No way! That just sounds sappy. I'm not comfortable writing a letter like that."), and for Phil and his wife to speak with their minister about marriage counseling ("Are you *kidding* me? I don't want the reverend to know our business!").

When it came to trying to manage his neck pain, Phil was encouraged to spend less time playing games on his smartphone, as looking down at his screen flattened the natural curve in his cervical spine, increasing pain. ("Seriously, you think *that's* the problem? I've had pain way longer than I've had a smartphone!") At his physical therapist's recommendation to take a five-minute stretching break every hour while at work to relax his muscles, decrease stress, and ease his sciatica, Phil just shook his head. "Do you have *any* idea of how busy my job is? I barely can remember to eat lunch or go to the bathroom."

In short, Phil was an expert at coming up with reasons why absolutely *nothing* would work. As a result, he continued to complain but refused to try anything new; thus, there was no improvement in his pain or his relationship. In essence, Phil's "crystal ball" was accurate in that he was "too far gone" to get better.

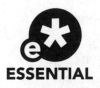

ESSENTIAL

If the Phil scenario sounds a bit familiar to you, or you have received feedback from friends and family that you tend to ask for help, reject most suggestions, and continue to struggle, a good therapist can help you try to break this pattern. It's worth remembering that changing a pattern or getting out of a rut begins with doing *even one thing* differently.

Anxiety

Anxiety has also been linked to greater disability, increased likelihood of medically unexplained symptoms, and decreased overall quality of life. People who have a chronic pain syndrome are more likely to be diagnosed as having panic, a phobia (possibly one related to a medical treatment), or social anxiety.

QUESTION

What is a phobia?
A phobia is an exaggerated, irrational fear of something. Patients who have significant dental pain may be phobic about visiting the dentist, and therefore avoid going for check ups or seeking treatment when a problem arises. This type of phobia can ultimately result in dental problems—and pain—becoming much worse.

One type of anxiety that you may have experienced is anticipatory anxiety, which refers to the act of worrying ahead of time that something will trigger or worsen either your pain or your anxiety. Sometimes people talk about the latter as "worrying about worrying." And whether you worry about triggering a pain increase or that you will become more anxious than you can bear, or both, worry can get in the way of doing things that have been important to you such as walking your child to school, playing a game of basketball, going to the movies, socializing with friends and family, eating certain foods, or even having sex. In fact, the worry can become so great that you may hesitate to leave your home at all, such as in the case of agoraphobia (fear of open spaces), social anxiety (anxiety related to being around others), and generalized anxiety disorder (where the anxiety feels more constant and the triggers are less obvious or circumscribed).

If you have suffered a trauma related to the cause of your pain, such as an automobile accident or serious injury, you may also have symptoms of something called posttraumatic stress disorder, or PTSD. Some of the symptoms of PTSD include hypervigilance, meaning that you are constantly hyperaware of your surroundings and on the lookout for something to go wrong; nightmares of the traumatic event; and intrusive, frightening thoughts that feel difficult to control. Whether you have a diagnosable condition or just find yourself feeling keyed up and on edge, anxiety issues can make it difficult to lead a life where you feel safe, happy, and able to do the things you need and want to.

As with depression, if you have been anxious for some time, or if you would describe yourself as someone who has always been a "worrier," it may be challenging to determine whether your feelings reflect what is generally "true" or whether you are suffering from a condition that requires treatment. The following are some of the symptoms of generalized anxiety:

SYMPTOMS OF GENERALIZED ANXIETY
- Ongoing worry that often is out of proportion or persists despite evidence that contradicts the worry
- Irritability
- Muscle tension
- Increased urination frequency
- Difficulty sleeping
- Feeling of "edginess"

In addition to what is referred to as generalized anxiety, you may experience feelings of panic, including tightness in the chest, rapid breathing, sweaty palms, rapid heartbeat, trembling, numbness or tingling, dizziness, and a sensation of or belief in impending catastrophe. If you experience a panic attack you can also experience feelings of "derealization," the sense of things being unreal somehow, or "depersonalization," the feeling of being outside yourself in some way. Other features common to a panic attack are the fear that you are "going crazy" or will die.

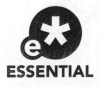

ESSENTIAL

Depression and anxiety are very real conditions that need to be evaluated and treated. Fear of being thought of as "crazy" prevents many people from seeking treatment that could alleviate symptoms and get them back to feeling more like themselves. Taking care of yourself when you are not feeling well is not only essential for good health and functioning but also very, very sane!

Symptoms of panic disorder can resemble those of a serious medical illness such as a thyroid problem, heart attack, or respiratory illness, resulting in visits to emergency rooms and doctors' offices. If you have had these symptoms, you should consult your healthcare provider promptly to rule out any physical illness. If your medical evaluation fails to confirm a physical health problem, the next step is to consult with a mental health professional who can evaluate you and help you take steps to feel better.

Like depression, anxiety can worsen the physical symptoms you may already have and can also lead to additional ones.

"Somatization" refers to the experience of emotions as bodily symptoms, including pain. This can happen in the form of headaches, digestive problems, joint or muscle pain, fatigue, or other sensations. If you hold in or deny strong feelings such as sadness, anger, fear, or grief, you may somaticize them, which can worsen the symptoms of an existing pain disorder or other health problem.

When You Should Seek Treatment

What follows are three questions to ask yourself that can help you determine whether your worry or sadness is something for which you should seek treatment:

- Do you feel sad or down, worried or fearful more of the time than not?
- Has your worry, fear, sadness, or hopelessness prevented you doing things you used to enjoy?
- Have the symptoms in the previous question prevented you functioning normally at work, at home, or in your relationships?

If you answered "yes" to any of these questions, it's worth contacting a licensed mental health professional in your area to help you understand what's fueling these feelings and develop the tools to feel better.

The Pros and Cons of Antidepressant Medications

If your pain has not responded to other medications or interventions, if you have had ongoing trouble sleeping, or if you have been experiencing symptoms of anxiety, depression, or both, your doctor may recommend "psychotropic" medications. These medications can include ones to help you feel calmer and less anxious, such as benzodiazepines, as well as medications prescribed purely to treat insomnia. Your doctor may also recommend you take an antidepressant medication, which can help not only with symptoms of depression such as sadness, difficulty concentrating or getting things done, and hopelessness but also with insomnia, feelings of anxiety, and pain severity.

There are several potential pros to taking a psychotropic medication. These include feeling less weighed down by your emotions, getting much-needed rest after battling insomnia, and feeling more able to get out into the world and do some of the things you may have been avoiding because your pain or mood have made them feel too difficult. Another pro is that after trying several medications for pain, once on the right antidepressant you may find that it enables you to replace several medications you have been taking separately to manage sleep, worry, depression, and pain.

The cons of taking any medication are that you may experience undesirable side effects such as dry mouth or decreased sexual desire, or you may try a medication and find it is not helpful at alleviating symptoms. In addition, any medication may interact with other conventional or complementary therapies you are using. Another significant con for many people is that taking an antidepressant may be at odds with a desire to use only "natural" substances as part of their treatment. This desire is certainly not a "wrong" one. But if you find that your CAM-only program still leaves you with pain and mood symptoms that prevent you feeling you can do the things you need and want to, it is worth discussing medication and other options with your pain specialist or a mental health professional.

Stigma and Antidepressants

Perhaps the greatest barrier to using psychotropic medications for pain is the stigma many people attach to them. Stigmas related to medication can be individual, such that someone who believes it's nonstigmatizing to take a benzodiazepine like Valium to help with feeling "keyed up" may be completely opposed to taking the antidepressant Zoloft for this purpose. Yet, benzodiazepines should not be used long term, in most cases (even though many people wind up taking them for months or years), and aren't considered the most effective medications if the goals are to both decrease symptoms of anxiety and prevent feelings of floatiness, disconnection, or sedation.

Relatedly, someone may feel completely comfortable taking the herb St. John's Wort to treat symptoms of depression, believing it to be risk-free because it is a natural substance. Yet, this remedy has some of the same side effects as antidepressant medications and can decrease the effectiveness of other medications like protease inhibitors (for patients with HIV) and warfarin (a drug to reduce blood clotting).

If the belief is that natural remedies are effective enough to help, it's important to be aware of their also being potentially potent enough to cause harm or interact with other herbs or drugs.

Why Antidepressants Are Prescribed for Pain

Your brain is complex, and the many areas of the brain involved in creating the experience of pain also play important roles in memory, thinking, planning, and judgment, as well as emotions such as depression. Some of the areas of the brain implicated in both pain and depression include the amygdala, hippocampus, thalamus, anterior cingulate, prefrontal cortical areas, and insular cortex.

It's no surprise, when you think about it, that medications targeting one aspect of brain functioning can impact others. In fact, sometimes a medication that does one thing is also specifically marketed for another purpose under a different name. This is because pharmaceutical companies are well aware that although you may feel uncomfortable with the idea of taking an antidepressant, you may not think twice about taking another kind of medication.

An example is the antidepressant Wellbutrin (buproprion). Buproprion is used to treat both major depression and seasonal depression, but the drug is also useful for smoking cessation. The drug Zyban is buproprion, just marketed under another name. Many people would say that taking Zyban is acceptable, but would hesitate to take Wellbutrin, not realizing that they are one and the same. Buproprion is sometimes prescribed to help manage both depression symptoms and pain.

Psychotropic medications are drugs that affect your mood, thinking, or behavior in some way. They are commonly prescribed to help with pain. In these cases, the "side effects"—sleepiness, or analgesia (pain relief)—are useful and desirable effects. If you choose to take a psychotropic medication for pain or mood, your doctor will advise you about the best dose and time to take it, and also about possible interactions with other medications, supplements, or alcohol.

Natural Mood Boosters

In the chapters on diet, supplements, CBT, mindfulness, hypnosis, exercise, biofeedback, and others, you will read more about nondrug remedies for anxiety and depression. Briefly, omega-3 fatty acids from fish, the supplement SAMe, and a healthy diet in general can improve symptoms of pain and depression, and help you cope better in general. Magnesium can have a mild calming effect and help with sleep issues. CBT, mindfulness, hypnosis, and biofeedback can be very valuable tools for managing anxiety and lessening depressive symptoms. Exercise is linked to better mood as well as to better memory, learning, and attention. The previous therapies will often have the greatest impact when used in some combination.

How Pain Can Impact Relationships

Pain is often poorly understood by those who have not had a chronic pain issue. You may have felt hard-pressed to explain to friends, family, and coworkers (and even to many healthcare providers) how your life has changed since developing chronic pain and why the experience is so distressing. A spouse or partner may become frustrated with the changes in your ability to perform household chores, desire for sexual intimacy, and mood changes. Friends may not understand why, months after a "successful surgery," since the cast was removed, or following your recovery from an illness, you continue to decline more social invitations than you accept. Your children may complain that you no longer play with them like you used to.

Communicating about Pain at Work

For many people, the most challenging place to communicate directly about pain is at work. Your boss, coworkers, or employees may doubt the validity of your absences for medical appointments. Fear of what others think of you may prompt you to overcompensate. You may find yourself taking on more responsibility, avoiding taking breaks, or seeking to hide your pain condition in some way to "make up" for the times when you can't perform as well as you did before developing chronic pain. Although understandable, this approach rarely works in the long run, and in fact can lead to an all or nothing pattern of performance—you are either "Superman" or "out of commission" with pain.

Kenny's Rollercoaster

After several months of unemployment, Kenny had started a new sales job and was working hard to impress his boss. Initially, he attempted to schedule medical and other appointments very early in the morning, or when his boss was out of town, but it had become more and more difficult to hide from everyone at work the fact that he had debilitating migraines.

"I worry that if I don't *overproduce* this quarter, it won't be enough to make up for all of the times I leave work—for the neurologist, or the acupuncturist, or for therapy. And maybe they will think I'm not serious about doing well here."

Kenny worried that the new job would lead to even more stress, which would potentially trigger more migraines, ultimately decrease his productivity, and jeopardize his job. In an attempt to stave off these feelings and ensure that his boss saw him as indispensable, Kenny found himself in a vicious cycle of trying to appear "normal," going the extra mile, and then needing several days to recover. When Kenny's boss asked him if he was okay, Kenny minimized his health issues and assured his boss he'd soon be "good as new."

Each time Kenny felt better, he resumed working long hours, sometimes missing meals. His stress increased, sleep quality decreased, and migraines became more frequent and harder to manage. After another marathon few weeks, Kenny once again had a migraine that kept him out of work for several days and led to his missing an important client meeting. Unaware of the severity of Kenny's migraines and not knowing much about this condition, Kenny's boss expressed the concern that Kenny didn't take his job seriously, or might simply be unreliable.

In the chapter on CBT, you will learn how Kenny (and anyone) could use pacing to get off the roller coaster at work, decrease stress, and probably have fewer severe pain episodes.

Indirect vs. Direct: Ways of Communicating about Pain

How you communicate with others is something you may take for granted. Speaking, writing, a gesture, touch, or a facial expression all say something to others about how you feel. If your communication isn't clear, however, it won't effectively get your point across and may even convey something different from what you intend.

How you communicate is influenced by a number of factors, including your temperament, such as how shy or outgoing you are. It can also be influenced by culture, gender, and how your family has responded to your speaking your mind, asking for help, or expressing feelings. In your relationships, you may be the person that everyone looks to for advice, or you may serve as a leader, and thus be quite accustomed to speaking frankly. If you grew up with the dictum, "Children should be seen and not heard," or "If you don't have anything nice to say, don't say anything at all," expressing yourself candidly may feel unthinkable. Similarly, if your family members were uncomfortable with the expression of emotions, or viewed illness as a sign of weakness, you may very well find it especially difficult to talk about pain. And if you have been the family caretaker, always meeting other people's needs, you may feel uncomfortable with the idea of asking others for assistance.

It's important to be aware of your natural communication style, however, because this will impact—for better or worse—how you let others know about your needs, wants, fears, and worries about pain—if you do so at all. Yet, communicating effectively is essential to good pain management, and if you don't communicate directly you may find some of your frustration lodges in your body, only to "speak up" as an increase in pain, fatigue, or sleep problems, etc.

"Cheryl the Caretaker"

Cheryl was a single mother in her late 40s with chronic fatigue and pain following surgery and radiation for breast cancer a few years prior. She had returned to work, but every day felt like a struggle. Her doctors had prescribed a variety of medicines but none seemed to help, leaving Cheryl discouraged and depressed. Cheryl also worried about how she was going to continue working and supporting her three adult children, all of whom still lived at home. On her doctor's advice, Cheryl attended a pain management group and received individual psychotherapy to learn nondrug approaches for pain relief. Each week, Cheryl complained that all three of her children worked but still asked her for money. None of them contributed to household expenses or helped her with chores, but they bought themselves expensive clothing and accessories and went out to eat when Cheryl was unable to cook for them.

Cheryl's pain, fatigue, and frustration seemed to increase each week, but when anyone asked Cheryl why she continued to support and clean up after her adult children, asking for nothing in return, she became angry and tearful. "I just *can't*," she'd say. "You don't understand—this is the way it's always been." Although many people tried to help Cheryl find her voice and set some new house rules, she felt unable to express her needs. On a few occasions, Cheryl said she had, in fact, asked her children to help with specific tasks, and told them that she needed them to contribute to household expenses.

"You know, it's really difficult for me to afford everything on my own . . . and I'm *so tired* today . . . it's hard to think of vacuuming right now . . . " Yet, things at home had not changed. The members of the pain management group encouraged her to be more direct, and the next week Cheryl reported that she had asked, "Hey, can you guys help around the house . . . when you get a chance? It's tough to manage on my own." To this, Cheryl's children said they had a number of "reasons" why they could not help her either practically or financially, and Cheryl felt discouraged, hopeless, and resentful.

"They'll help me only when I get so sick that I can't do anything anymore!" she said. As Cheryl's distress increased, so did her pain. Cheryl eventually took a medical leave from her job and stopped coming for group therapy. It's not known whether her children finally pitched in, moved out, or continued doing things in exactly the same way.

In Cheryl's case, she had always demonstrated her love for her children and others in her life by pampering them and asking nothing in return. Because she had put her needs last (or denied she even had them), her now adult children had never learned to either be fully self-sufficient or consider that she, like they, had needs. It was understandable that Cheryl, after a lifetime of avoiding frank discussions, setting limits, or asking for anything would feel unable to express herself directly and stand her ground.

Making this significant a change would absolutely be challenging, and most likely, Cheryl would have needed a good deal of support and guidance in order for her efforts to be successful. In the absence of this level of support and commitment, many people like Cheryl find that their distress gets shoved down inside them, and their physical symptoms worsen. The pain ultimately winds up doing the talking for them.

Indirect Communication

Indirect communication can serve a number of purposes, and many times, the purpose may not even be one that you are fully conscious of at the time you "say" something. Whatever your communication style, chronic pain may intensify your tendency to default to the mode of communication that feels most natural for you. But it may not be the most effective way to express yourself and help others understand what you need. What many people have difficulty realizing is that being indirect can make it much harder for others to be honest with you about what kind of support they feel able to offer, because the unspoken message is, being direct is not okay—for either of you.

Do you default to any of these indirect ways of being?

"The Hero"

The Hero is very stoical and tries hard to pretend he is not only not in pain, but is as good as ever! He is saying, "It's essential that you think I am fine, because it's not permissible for me to be vulnerable, weak, in pain, or 'needy.' I must appear strong at all times." As a result, the person with this theme may be less likely to follow up with important doctor's appointments or may overdo strenuous activities. Although this style of communication may preserve the Hero's need to feel and appear superhuman for a while, his failure to pace himself and get proper care could backfire, leading to worse pain and greater vulnerability down the road. Taking on this role may very well preserve others' beliefs in the Hero's superhuman powers for a time, but they may ultimately feel blindsided and unprepared for his "sudden" symptoms and need for help if his condition worsens.

"The Silent Film Star"

This person communicates pain or the need for assistance by wincing, bracing, guarding a tender body part, or sharply sucking in her breath. Oftentimes, when someone is in pain they will evidence some sort of pain behavior, but the silent film star tends to exaggerate these gestures. What she is communicating with her body, but not her voice, is, "I really want your help with this, but I am afraid you will say 'no' or think badly of me if I ask you directly. If I *show* you how bad I feel, maybe you will finally understand how serious this is and help me. I really hope you notice . . . " This style of communication, while sometimes effective at eliciting concern and care from others, can also backfire—it can leave those around her feeling that the silent film star is simply acting.

"The Orchestrator"

The orchestrator acknowledges having a pain condition and consciously lets the pain do the talking and limit setting—at times, even when the pain is under control. Thus, the headache, back pain, or fatigue may be referenced or invoked as a way to end an unpleasant conversation, make a demand for care, or avoid engaging in specific activities—even when the symptoms feel fairly manageable. The communication is, "I don't want you to refuse my request or expect me to do something that I'd rather not. And I *definitely* don't want to talk about any issues." In a sense, the pain can serve as the Orchestrator's weapon, shield, and negotiation tool.

Members of the Orchestrator's primary support group may struggle both with resentment about his constant demands and the guilt that this type of communication induces in them. Although many people will initially say "yes" because the Orchestrator suffers from something painful, they may ultimately avoid dealing with him whenever possible.

"The Smiler"

When anxious or uncomfortable about something, the Smiler's facial expression, tone of voice, or both will be incongruent, or different, from the emotional tone of what she is saying. Often, the Smiler is unaware of this tendency and will continue to smile, laugh, or otherwise negate in some way the message she is consciously trying to get across. This happens especially when describing something distressing, asking for help that she believes she won't receive, or attempting to have an emotionally frank conversation that she believes the other person won't be receptive to.

It's as though a part of the Smiler wants to be understood, but another part feels unentitled, like what she is saying is inappropriate because it's related to a problem, or that she will be judged or rejected as a result of the communication. The smiling is unconsciously designed to "take back" the part of the communication that the Smiler believes will cause the problem. In some instances, it may seem like this form of disowning or negating whatever is unpleasant softens the blow of challenging or uncomfortable information for either the Smiler, the recipient of the message, or both of them, but very often this tendency leaves others confused or doubting the truth or validity of the Smiler's message—or even doubting the Smiler's general sincerity.

Effective Communication

Because chronic pain can force changes in the role you play in your relationships, or bring challenges to the surface, it can generate fears and questions about who you are now that you have pain. These changes can trigger feelings of grief, sadness, and anxiety. You may also fear that you will no longer be lovable or acceptable if you are not your "old self." It is normal to fear or resent the changes that pain brings about. And it's also normal to fear that others won't relate to you in the same way due to the changes pain makes in your life.

These particular fears can make it feel even more challenging to communicate directly. In the long run, communicating indirectly can lead to more problems than it solves. Learning to communicate effectively, although it may take some practice in the beginning, will have benefits that extend beyond simply talking about pain.

Direct Communication

Many people avoid communicating directly because they believe it is equivalent to being aggressive or demanding. Yet effective communication is both direct in that the intended meaning is clear to both the communicator and the person hearing the message, and is also respectful of both parties. It leaves room for each person involved to be honest and to have her own opinion. Furthermore, effective communication acknowledges that each party has challenges, needs, wants, and strengths, and that arriving at a solution may take some work and compromise on everyone's parts.

What Effective Communication Is Not

Effective communication is not about being aggressive, nor is it about being the loudest person in the room. It's also not about ensuring that other people always agree with you or comply with your wishes, even though it's normal to hope that they will—at least some of the time. Furthermore, effective communication is definitely not about attempting to manipulate, sweet talk, or trick others into doing things for you, whether out of pity, guilt, or obligation. And certainly, communicating effectively is not about working so hard to avoid stressing or inconveniencing others that your own needs never get met.

Communicating effectively is, in a sense, one way of investing in the integrity of a relationship. It sets a standard for the present as well as for the future. You may also notice that as you become more aware of your own effort to communicate effectively about pain and in general, you may become more appreciative of others' efforts to do the same—and less patient with others' attempts to communicate indirectly.

SOME RULES FOR EFFECTIVE COMMUNICATION ABOUT PAIN
- Use "I statements" to talk about feelings, needs, and wants: "I feel frustrated about XYZ and want to see if we can reach a compromise," not "You caused me to feel . . . ," which tends to shut down communication and unfairly make the other person responsible for your emotional reaction.
- Don't assume others know what you need, understand how you are feeling, or know how "helping you" would look exactly.
- Be *specific* and *concrete* about what you need help with, such as, "Please help me carry this bag of groceries," or "I'd like you to babysit on Wednesdays if you are available," instead of "You need to help me out more."

- Distinguish between "wants" and "needs." Prioritize those things that require help and need to be done first, understanding that you may not get everything you want, but you will hopefully receive more assistance with needs.
- To get your point across, "Strike when the iron is *cold*." In other words, wait until you and the other person are both calm before initiating communication about emotionally sensitive topics.
- Stay focused in the here and now of the relationship rather than bringing in previous examples of when someone failed to be helpful.
- Talk about the behavior, if you are discussing a problem, or what you would specifically like to see change, rather than seek to change another's feelings, desires, or personality (you won't be successful at changing these anyway).
- Avoid generalizations or labeling the other person as the problem ("You are uncaring."). Frame in terms of the positives of the desired action ("I appreciate when you help with the cleaning/come with me to doctors' appointments/notice how hard I am trying. It makes it easier to manage doing these things.").
- Try to avoid using "always" and "never" when bringing up a problem or issue ("You always dismiss my pain." or "You never help me.") as this tends to shut down the lines of communication. Plus, absolutes like "always" and "never" are likely inaccurate.
- Strive for balance between speaking and listening.
- Strive for congruence between what you are saying and your facial expressions, tone, and body language.

Understand that no amount of effective communication may make others understand what you are experiencing, feel comfortable talking about pain or illness, or make the changes you hope they will.

CHAPTER 5

Your Pain Management Team

Ideally, you will find that the medical members of your team are not only knowledgeable about the neurobiology and biomechanics of pain but also understand that pain causes significant distress. In addition, the right provider will be able to recommend other professionals outside his field, such as physical therapists, psychotherapists, or dieticians, who can further enhance your treatment. The best pain providers should help you create the regimen that helps you manage your symptoms and improve your functioning—even if your functioning does not return to what it was prior to your pain.

Choosing the Players on Your Team

One of the most important stress reducers you may experience is feeling you have found the "right players" for your pain management team. Putting a good team together can seem like a daunting process, particularly when you may already feel increased stress and less energy than normal. In addition, geographical location, insurance, and your finances may strongly influence the doctors you see and whether or not your team includes CAM providers, whose fees are less likely to be covered by insurance. That said, although the pain team will probably evolve as you learn what works and what doesn't for you with regard to therapies and treatment philosophies, you will benefit in the long run by taking the time to research potential team members ahead of time.

The Primary Care Physician

Even though your pain management team will be, of course, pain specific with regard to most of the players, you will likely want to continue seeing your primary care physician (PCP) or internist. Your PCP will be able to liaise with your pain professionals and address any other general health conditions or symptoms that arise, and may also be a good resource for finding out about other providers who may be useful additions to your team.

Another advantage of having a good PCP is that she may have known you for some time and will recognize changes in your physical or emotional well-being more readily than other doctors who have met you more recently. In addition, your specialist physicians will typically send a copy of their findings and lab results to your PCP after each visit. This will help you have all your information related to your pain condition in one place.

ESSENTIAL

If you need to find a new PCP, useful resources include the American Academy of Family Physicians (*www.familydoctor.org*) and the American Board of Internal Medicine (*www.abim.org*). To find a holistically inclined PCP, visit the Academy of Integrative Health & Medicine (formerly The American Holistic Medical Association; *http://aihm.org/find-a-provider*).

Pain Medicine Specialists

Depending on both your health issue and the type of conventional treatment you are seeking, your primary pain physician's medical specialty may be neurology, neurosurgery, anesthesiology, rehabilitation medicine, physical medicine, or orthopedics. If you seek treatment at a university or hospital-based pain center, you will also have access to other members of their pain management faculty, which can include nurses and nurse practitioners, physical therapists, psychologists or social workers, a dietitian, and perhaps a health educator. The table explains the differences between the various types of pain management doctors.

TYPES OF PAIN MANAGEMENT PHYSICIANS

Specialist	What They Do
Neurologist	Treats diseases of the nervous system, including the brain, spine, and nerves.
Neurosurgeon	Trained in surgery of the nervous system, including the brain, spine, and nerves themselves.
Anesthesiologist	Trained to prescribe or administer a range of medications and perform some procedures to treat pain. Also administers general and local anesthesia for a wide range of medical procedures, from dental to other surgical ones.
Orthopedist	Trained in evaluating and treating injuries and diseases of the musculoskeletal system, including bone and joint disorders.
Physiatrist	Trained to diagnose, treat, and prevent disease. Uses physical medicine—manipulation, massage, and exercise—to treat painful and nonpainful conditions.

When considering a pain physician, here are some good rules of thumb:

- Verify that the provider has completed a pain medicine fellowship that is accredited by the Accreditation Council for Graduate Medical Education (ACGME)
- In addition to having completed a pain medicine fellowship, verify that she is also board certified by visiting the American Board of Medical Specialties (*www.abms.org*)
- Select a provider who has a good reputation in your community. Ask your internist for his recommendations, and consult friends, family, and colleagues regarding their thoughts, if you are comfortable doing so

Once you have decided to consult with a specific doctor, here are additional criteria for finding the right fit:

- The provider should take the time to do a thorough initial intake and examination before recommending a treatment plan
- She should be able to discuss both short-term and long-term approaches to managing your pain
- He should be receptive to your questions regarding your health issue and the treatment plan proposed
- She or another member of the treatment team should be able to answer your questions as they arise, including after the initial consultation, by phone or e-mail
- Your doctor or a member of his team should return your non-emergency call by phone within one business day (two at most) unless there are extenuating circumstances
- He should be open to using a multimodal approach that may consist of medications, injections or other procedures, and physical therapy
- She should be able to explain how proposed medications or other treatments work and also discuss their limitations
- Your doctor should explain the potential risks and benefits to recommended treatments as well as alternatives to these
- She should be somewhat knowledgeable about the science with regard to CAM therapies for your particular condition, even if she does not provide them
- He should be willing to consult with your primary care provider and other members of your medical team, including your psychotherapist, physical or occupational therapist, dietitian, and other licensed or certified professionals, if applicable

FACT

Contrary to popular belief, there is no one type of "pain doctor." Physicians who work with pain should be trained and board certified in a specific subspecialty, such as neurology, anesthesiology, rehabilitation medicine, or psychiatry, and then have obtained formal postgraduate training in pain management.

Some clinics may also employ CAM providers such as a medical massage therapist, an acupuncturist, or even a yoga instructor, but CAM therapists are still the exception rather than the rule in these settings.

Questions to Ask Regarding Insurance

Discussing the financial aspect of the doctor-patient relationship can feel awkward, but for most people it's essential to assess beforehand whether you can afford the provider you are hoping to see. Developing a comfortable rapport with a doctor only to feel blindsided by a large bill—especially if it's out of your budget—will only add extra stress, which is certainly not a great thing for pain management. Here are some tips for taking the stress out of the process:

- Call well ahead of time to see if the provider participates in your insurance plan. If so, ask what the copay will be for the visit.
- If your provider is out-of-network, ask what the fee is for the consultation.
- Contact your insurer to see if you have out-of-network benefits. If so, ask the amount of your deductible and whether you have met it.
- Ask the insurance contact how much of the consultation fee charged will be covered. If the answer is, "We cover 60 percent of reasonable and customary," ask specifically what amount they consider "reasonable and customary."
- Determine whether you can realistically afford whatever amount will not be covered by your insurance plan.

Factor into the estimated costs that you will likely see your pain provider several times per year, particularly if your pain is not yet under control, if the provider prescribes medication for you, or if she will be performing a procedure of some sort.

Preparing for Your First Appointment

All doctors will differ somewhat with regard to what they find most helpful in terms of background information. A good rule of thumb is to ask the receptionist (or check the practice website) to see what they request. Here are a few other tips to help you get the most out of your first appointment:

- If possible, send copies of laboratory and physician reports (keep originals for your records) by mail or fax a week before your first appointment
- Even if you have faxed or mailed copies of your reports, bring hard copies to the consultation, just in case
- Bring copies of films from diagnostic procedures, if you have them
- Write down and bring a list of up to five of your most pressing questions, noted in order of priority
- Write down your current list of medications and assess which ones will need to be refilled within the next month
- Have the name and phone number of your pharmacy on hand
- Have a list of all current healthcare providers, with their contact information
- Be frank and specific when describing your symptoms
- Let your doctor know about any adverse reactions you have had to any medications, pain-related or otherwise
- Be frank about any issues related to taking pain medicine, including any history of substance dependence or abuse

Some practices will provide intake forms online or e-mail these to you prior to your first visit; others may not. But the more organized and concise you can be with regard to providing important information about your health in general and pain, specifically, the more data your doctor will have on hand to determine what might be the most helpful approach for you. In addition, being organized will enable you and your doctor to use the time available most efficiently.

The pre-consultation questionnaire that follows can help you to have some important information at the ready for your first meeting with a new provider.

Pre-Consultation Questionnaire

1. Where are you experiencing pain?

    _____

    _____

    _____

2. Please indicate which areas have been painful for 3 months or more.

    _____

    _____

3. Please indicate, for each painful condition, when it began, and if known, what triggered it (e.g., headaches following childbirth, pain following an accident, etc.).

Condition	When Started	Trigger

4. Please circle all of the terms that describe your most prominent pain:

Sharp	Stinging	Pounding
Throbbing	Intermittent	Constant
Electrical	Aching	Stabbing
Hot	Cutting	Tight
Squeezing	Crushing	Tugging
Dull	Burning	Itchy
Radiating	Severe	Mild
Moderate		

5. If there is more than one, which painful area is most bothersome to you?

_____

_____

6. On a scale of zero to ten, with zero indicating no pain at all, and ten indicating the worst possible pain, please rate the following:

Your average level of pain in the past week _____
Your highest pain rating in the past week _____
Your lowest pain rating in the past week _____

7. Have you ever seen another doctor to manage the painful condition(s) listed here? If so, please provide the dates, names, and contact information for each doctor, as well as their area of specialization (e.g., neurologist, psychiatrist, internist, chiropractor, other health professional).

Dates   Provider Name and contact information   Specialization

_____

_____

8. Please indicate the treatments you have tried for pain management, including if they were helpful.

Medications tried: Who prescribed them?   Which were helpful?

_____

_____

9. If you discontinued a medication, please indicate which and why.

_____

_____

10. Procedures or surgeries for pain: Please list and indicate if they were help-
    ful or not.

    _____

    _____

11. Devices (e.g., TENS): Please list and indicate if they were helpful or not.

    _____

    _____

12. Have you engaged in physical therapy? If so, please include the dates and
    whether this was helpful to you.

    _____

    _____

13. Which complementary or alternative medicine (CAM) treatments have
    you tried? (Please circle)

Herbal remedies	Dietary Supplements	Special Diets
Movement therapies (yoga, tai chi, etc.)	Energy Healing	Meditation
Hypnosis/Guided imagery	Acupuncture	Massage
Traditional Medical Systems (Chinese medicine, Ayurveda, etc.)	Homeopathy	

14. Please list other CAM treatments you have tried that are not mentioned
    here:

    _____

    _____

15. What complementary or alternative treatments are you using currently?

_____

_____

16. Using a zero to ten scale, where zero means no support at all, and ten means feeling the best social support possible, please indicate your current level of social support:

_____

_____

17. Which medications are you taking currently? Please list even if you are not taking them to address pain (e.g., antidepressants, cholesterol lowering drugs, medications for anxiety or sleep, etc.).

_____

_____

18. Please describe your current exercise habits, including the type, frequency, and duration.

_____

_____

19. Please briefly describe your regular diet.

_____

_____

20. How many servings of caffeine (coffee, tea, soda) do you drink per day? (Note: consider a serving to be an 8-oz glass.)

_____

_____

21. How many alcoholic beverage servings do you consume per week, on average? (Note: a serving is 12 ounces, or one can of beer, 5 ounces of wine, or 1.5 ounces of hard liquor—whiskey, vodka, gin, etc.).

_____

_____

22. Do you smoke? If so, please indicate how many cigarettes per day.

_____

If you answered "yes" to the previous question, please indicate how many years you have been smoking.

_____

23. Please list any other health problems you have.

_____

_____

24. Have you ever been treated for a mental health issue?

_____

_____

25. If "yes," please indicate the issue(s) and whether you are in treatment currently.

_____

_____

26. Have you ever tried cognitive-behavioral therapy to manage your pain? Would you be receptive to trying this approach?

_____

_____

27. Please list any recreational drugs you take, even occasionally.

_____

_____

28. How are you hoping the provider can help you?

_____

_____

29. Are you willing to make lifestyle changes (e.g., quitting smoking, changing diet, getting exercise, practicing relaxation techniques) if this could help your pain?

_____

_____

30. What factors help your pain to decrease?

   _____

   _____

31. What factors seem to worsen your pain?

   _____

   _____

32. Please use the space here to write about anything else you think your provider should know about your chronic pain or health in general.

   _____

   _____

When to Switch Pain Doctors

Finding the right pain doctor or clinic can feel challenging, and as stated earlier in the chapter, you may feel your choices are somewhat limited due to your geographical location, insurance coverage, or finances. Furthermore, in some areas there may be few (or perhaps only one) specialists formally trained in pain management. But within the parameters you have, it's important to feel that you have some choice, if possible.

Doctors are People, Too

It may seem obvious, but oftentimes patients can forget that doctors are people, too, who have good days and bad, have skills and challenges, are vulnerable to personal illnesses, and can be occasionally insensitive or forgetful when stressed or busy. If you are like a good number of people who have been dealing with chronic pain for some time, you have probably encountered providers you have found helpful and lovely to be around, those who have been helpful but lacked a degree of interpersonal sensitivity, those who have been not so helpful but nice to be around, and those who have seemed both unhelpful and not terribly enjoyable.

Sometimes, even the "A+" providers may have a bad day, seem a bit harried, forget a detail if your chart is not right in front of them, take longer than normal to respond to a non-urgent phone call, or run unusually late. And there is probably no provider who will know everything about every possible treatment for your condition (particularly when it comes to CAM therapies). When all is said and done, you should use your own judgment with regard to whether to continue a relationship with a provider—CAM or conventional. Here are some guidelines to help you decide whether to "take the bad with the good" or find a new provider:

WHEN TO STAY WITH YOUR PROVIDER

- Your doctor meets reasonable criteria with regard to training, board certification, postgraduate education in pain management, and ongoing professional involvement in the field of pain (e.g., belonging to pain-related professional associations)
- He listens to your questions and communicates with respect
- She is reasonably on time most of the time
- The office appears clean and the office staff is polite and helpful
- Your pain is improving or is at least more tolerable
- If your pain has not yet improved, your doctor is willing to work to try to find a more helpful approach
- Your doctor seems up-to-date regarding recent scientific developments related to your condition
- He clearly explains the potential risks and benefits of proposed treatments
- You receive a return phone call within forty-eight hours at most about non-urgent matters
- Your dissatisfaction, if any, is with the office staff rather than the doctor

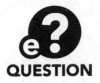

QUESTION

What is board certification, and why should my doctor be board certified?
Board certification goes beyond medical licensure and verifies that your doctor has met nationally recognized standards for education, knowledge, experience, and skills for a specific medical specialty. You can see if your physician is board certified by going to the American Board of Medical Specialties website: *http://certificationmatters.org*.

WHEN TO FIND ANOTHER DOCTOR

- You feel your concerns are typically dismissed or invalidated
- He is more than thirty minutes late more often than not
- Your doctor frequently forgets your name or primary health problem
- Your pain has not improved and your doctor is out of ideas about how to help you
- Your doctor dismisses the possibility you might benefit from a treatment with which he is admittedly unfamiliar
- Your doctor does not seem to know much about your particular medical condition or the standards for treating it
- Your doctor does not explain why she is recommending a particular treatment
- He does not explain the potential risks and benefits of a recommended treatment
- More than once or twice, you have not received a return phone call within forty-eight hours related to non-urgent medical issues
- The office is dirty, or the doctor or staff does not follow standard practices related to hygiene or sanitizing of equipment
- Your doctor is opposed to or offended by your seeking a second opinion
- Your doctor is defensive or aggressive when you bring concerns to his attention
- Your doctor is not board certified in his area of specialization
- Your doctor has no formal postgraduate training in pain management

Sometimes, whether you stay with a particular provider will come down to other factors such as geographic location, ease of getting to the office, or if your insurance reimburses for her services. One of the most influential factors may be difficult to define, but you will know it when you feel it: an overall level of comfort with and trust in your provider that may make all the difference.

How "Expert" Is Your Expert?

It's not always easy to tell how much your doctor knows about your specific medical issue, as "pain management" can encompass treating a wide variety of conditions, some of which will be more common than others. Although a provider's level of expertise will not guarantee that you will either feel comfortable with or have the desired results with her, it will tell you something about what she may know about working with pain in general and your issue in particular.

One way to assess your doctor's involvement in the field of pain management is to see whether she is a member of any regional, national, or international pain societies such as the Eastern Pain Association, the American Pain Society, or the International Association for the Study of Pain. Your provider may also belong to a professional association that focuses on a specific type of pain, such as the American Headache Society.

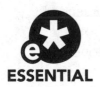

ESSENTIAL

The International Association for the Study of Pain (IASP) provides links to over thirty other professional associations related to chronic pain. You can view this list on their website: *www.iasp-pain.org*. In addition, you may wish to contact the American Board of Pain Medicine (*www .abpm.org*) to find a formally trained pain management provider.

You may also wish to see whether your doctor has published scientific articles related to pain. You can find this out by using PubMed, a free, government-funded search engine that enables you to find the titles and abstracts of scientific articles by topic or author. Visiting *www.ncbi.nlm.nih .gov/pubmed/* and typing in your doctor's first and last name should show you if he has published at all, and if so, whether within the field of pain.

You will probably notice that doctors who are affiliated with universities or teaching hospitals are more likely to have engaged in and published findings from their research. Of course, having a scholarly background does not guarantee a doctor will be the right fit for you or have a good bedside manner. Similarly, a provider may be knowledgeable and competent but not have published in the pain-related scientific literature. But your provider should be able to demonstrate an interest and ongoing involvement in the field of pain management beyond seeing patients who present with chronic pain.

If you are not located near enough to a pain specialist to see one regularly, determine whether your internist is willing to liaise with a pain specialist of your choosing (and who will have evaluated you in person) in order to coordinate care. Certain medications or procedures will only be provided via your pain physician, but your regular doctor may be able to provide monitoring and order more routine blood work and imaging in the interim.

Community Members As Team Members

Because chronic pain can be an isolating and uniquely challenging experience, and because doctors and family may have limited time (and sometimes limited training) to offer emotional support, it's important to have part of your team consist of people who understand the pain experience from a personal perspective.

One resource that can help you connect with others who have the same or a similar pain syndrome is Friends Health Connection. This organization was founded in the late 1980s by a young woman, Roxanne Black, who was diagnosed with lupus. Roxanne wanted to find support from another person who was both a similar age and understood the experience of having lupus from a personal perspective. What began as one-on-one support has now grown into a thriving national network. The website offers ways to obtain support and also features video and audio inspirational and educational talks by well-known speakers, including Dr. Bernie Siegel, Dr. Larry Dossey, and His Holiness the Dalai Lama. To learn more, visit *www .friendshealthconnection.org*.

CAM Providers

The field of integrative medicine is incredibly broad, and the myriad specialties that fall under the CAM umbrella can have wide-ranging standards for certification or licensure. In addition, many therapies may not have a formal system of credentialing practitioners. For some therapies, the criteria for regulating and credentialing CAM specialists vary from state to state.

In general, state and local governments are responsible for deciding what credentials practitioners must have to work in their jurisdiction. It's worth noting that credentialing will not guarantee that a provider—conventional or CAM—is competent or will be able to help you specifically. The NCCIH clarifies different types of credentialing as well as provides some information about the CAM therapies that require it (e.g., chiropractic and naturopathy). To learn more, visit: *https://nccih.nih.gov/health/decisions/credentialing.htm*.

Selecting a CAM Therapy

The number of individual CAM therapies seems to be ever growing, and it is not possible to list them all here in this book. If you are new to including CAM in your treatment plan, it may be helpful ask yourself the following key questions:

- What am I hoping to address or achieve with CAM? (Enhanced relaxation? Greater muscle flexibility? Spiritual connectedness?)
- How active or passive do I want my participation in the therapy to be? (Do I want to be moving during the treatment? Resting? Am I interested in learning a new practice? Am I willing to devote time to the therapy process outside of actual sessions?)
- What is my budget for CAM? (Unlimited? Minimal? None at all?)
- Am I seeking therapy that is hands on? Hands off?
- Do I want to expand my social world (via classes, groups, or practice circles), or do I prefer one-on-one interaction?

These questions can help you get a better sense of what types of therapies may or may not be the right fit for you. This is particularly important as you may have had a number of well-intentioned friends or family suggest a wide range of CAM treatments (or alternatively, advocated against one in particular, or even CAM therapies in general).

After asking yourself these questions, it's also useful to be aware of the different, broad categories of CAM therapies. Some specific therapies may fall under more than one heading, such as Qigong (it's a movement-based therapy, but also an energy healing practice).

Types of CAM Therapies

- Dietary Systems (vegan, macrobiotic, Mediterranean); Traditional Healing Systems (Ayurveda, Traditional Chinese Medicine)
- Alternative Medical Systems (chiropractic, naturopathy, osteopathy); Manipulative Treatments (massage, reflexology, Rolfing)
- Movement-Based Therapies (yoga, Pilates, Qigong); Energy Therapies (Qigong, homeopathy, Healing Touch)
- Mind-Body Therapies (meditation, hypnosis, biofeedback); Spiritual Healing (intercessory prayer, prayer for one's own health)
- Use of Dietary Supplements (herbs, macronutrients, vitamins/minerals); "Superfoods" (green tea, pomegranate, spirulina)
- Psychological Approaches (cognitive-behavioral therapy, support groups, art therapy); Other approaches (music therapy, aromatherapy)

This list is necessarily brief and excludes many of the therapies you may have heard of, both due to space limitations as well as because some, like acupuncture, fall under the heading of Traditional Chinese Medicine. Both the key questions mentioned earlier in this section and this table can help get you started on your quest to find the right therapies for you.

FACT

NCCIH provides a list of six tips for finding the right CAM practitioner for you. You can access it here: *https://nccih.nih.gov/health/tips/selecting*. NCCIH also maintains an extensive list of CAM therapies and related topics, available online: *https://nccih.nih.gov/health/atoz.htm*. Finally, they maintain a list of clinical trials of CAM therapies that are currently recruiting participants: *https://clinicaltrials.gov*. At this writing, a large number of these are trials exploring the use of CAM therapies to treat chronic pain.

CHAPTER 6

Nutrition

You may be wondering what nutrition could possibly have to do with pain management. After all, food is not a drug or a remedy in the conventional sense. Yet both the research and anecdotal evidence suggest that the best diets in general emphasize unprocessed foods, and primarily fruits, vegetables, whole grains, and fish. Eating in this way can improve your mood, decrease the inflammation associated with many medical conditions, including pain, and increase general well-being. It's also worth noting that many, many people use food as a multipurpose tool—often to address cravings for comfort or distract from unpleasant emotions, in addition to fueling the body. Since poor eating habits can lead to over- or under-weight, and each of these can worsen pain and coping, it's worth taking a closer look at what you eat, how much, and why you eat the way you do.

Diet as a Pain Management Tool

There has been a bit of debate as to how certain foods may impact pain. Both some research and anecdotal evidence have found that avoiding some foods and incorporating others may impact uncomfortable symptoms. This is particularly true for those suffering from conditions such as migraines, pelvic pain, rheumatoid arthritis, and irritable bowel syndrome or other gastrointestinal illnesses.

The most conservative route is to strive to follow general guidelines for healthy nutrition. That is not bad advice or an incorrect stance to take. Another approach is to be even more deliberate with regard to investigating which foods worsen your pain, digestion, mood, or energy levels, as well as those that tend to help you feel better. As you pay more attention to what you eat and drink, and how you feel before and after, you will likely discover your own invaluable "data" about what dietary changes are most important for your good health. What follows are overall recommendations for a healthy, anti-inflammatory diet as well as a glimpse of some dietary adjustments shown to be helpful for specific conditions.

Reducing Inflammation and Improving Health

As mentioned previously, inflammation is a key factor in a number of medical illnesses, including chronic pain conditions. A pro-inflammatory diet may increase pain, decrease energy, stress the immune system, and increase the risk of illnesses like cancer and heart disease. Some pro-inflammatory foods are trans fats (also known as partially hydrogenated oils); sugar and corn syrup, as well as beverages made from these; processed carbohydrates such as those found in crackers, pie crusts, and cookies; and processed meats such as cold cuts. In general, processed foods offer little to no nutritional value other than calories and can make you feel worse than you need to. Anti-inflammatory foods include fatty fish, fruits, and vegetables in as close to their natural state as possible, eggs fortified with omega-3 fatty acids (listed as DHA on the carton), walnuts, and the like.

FACT

Simple food swaps can help you decrease your intake of pro-inflammatory foods without feeling deprived. They can also help you lose weight if you need to. An example: Two slices (31 g) of cheddar cheese have about 160 calories and 14 grams of fat, mostly saturated (and pro-inflammatory). One-fifth of an avocado (30 g) has about 50 calories and 5 grams of fat, mostly unsaturated.

EASY, ANTI-INFLAMMATORY FOOD SWAPS

Instead of this	Try this	Comment
¼ cup of croutons	½ cup cubed beets roasted in ½ teaspoon olive oil	The croutons have about 46 calories for this tiny amount, no fiber, and are loaded with refined carbohydrates. The beets drizzled with oil have 60 calories total (for twice the food) and contain healthy fats, 2 grams of fiber, vitamins, and antioxidants.
Hamburger (3 ounces)	Salmon (3 ounces)	The same size serving of salmon has 175 vs. 245 calories found in hamburger, a comparable amount of protein, mostly unsaturated fat, and is rich in omega-3 fatty acids.
Wheat crackers	Apple slices	For each serving of about 16 thin crackers, you would consume 140 calories of refined starch and hidden sugars. One medium apple has about 95 calories, water, fiber, and about 14 percent of the recommended daily amount of vitamin C.
12-ounce can of soda	Sparkling water with 1 ounce of pomegranate juice	The soda contains about 136 calories of sugar and unhealthy chemicals. Sparking water has no sugar or chemicals, hydrates your body, and the pomegranate juice has 17 calories, no harmful chemicals, and contains antioxidant polyphenols.
Milk chocolate	Dark chocolate	Milk chocolate is nutrient-poor and simply a source of fat, sugar, and calories. Dark chocolate is also fat and calorie-dense but is a good source of antioxidants and has been found to lower blood pressure. Aim for at least 70 percent dark.

Examples of Illness-Specific Dietary Changes

In addition to following a generally healthy and anti-inflammatory diet, many people with rheumatoid arthritis (RA) report benefit from avoiding foods in the nightshade family such as potatoes, tomatoes, eggplant, peppers, and tobacco (the latter you should avoid anyway). Others note no difference in symptoms from eliminating these foods. Similarly, many people with RA and other autoimmune conditions or gastrointestinal (GI) disorders report easing of symptoms from the avoidance of either wheat alone or any gluten-containing foods, even in the absence of a diagnosis of celiac disease. Certainly, many patients with Crohn's disease and other GI ailments find their pain and diarrhea are decreased if they eat cooked, rather than raw vegetables and limit intake of nuts, seeds, spicy foods, and caffeine.

Interstitial cystitis is another chronic pain condition that is responsive to dietary changes. Citrus fruits, tomatoes, vitamin C, artificial sweeteners, coffee, tea, carbonated and alcoholic beverages, and spicy foods can exacerbate symptoms. Conversely, there is some evidence that sodium bicarbonate (baking soda) tends to improve symptoms.

For those who suffer from migraines, under-eating, eating too infrequently, dehydration, and consuming certain foods can trigger migraines. The foods most commonly reported as triggers are alcohol (in general, and red wine specifically), caffeine, cheese, chocolate, and monosodium glutamate.

ALERT

Emulsifiers are common food additives that give foods a smooth and stable consistency. A recent study published in the journal *Nature* found that mice given two popular ones, CMC and polysorbate 80, had increased inflammation, became obese, and developed blood sugar issues. Genetically vulnerable mice were also more likely to develop inflammatory bowel disease from consuming these additives. So it's worth reducing intake of processed foods and these additives specifically.

With regard to pelvic pain, some research has shown that eating foods high in omega-3 fatty acids, magnesium, vitamin E, vitamin B_1, and vitamin B_3 can reduce the production of prostaglandins. Prostaglandins are chemicals in your body that increase inflammation, uterine cramping, and pain. A mainly plant-based diet of fruits, vegetables, nuts, and fish is higher in fiber and nutrients. In addition, diets that emphasize including healthy foods tend to naturally lead to lower consumption of refined sugars and processed fats that contribute to inflammation. With regard to fiber, dietary fiber intake is linked to a decrease in excess body fat and therefore results in lower levels of circulating estrogen (because fat cells produce estrogen). Decreasing circulating estrogen can limit the overgrowth of endometrial tissue associated with endometriosis, a cause of pelvic pain.

Again, although the chronic pain conditions covered here represent only a small sampling of those that may be impacted one way or the other by diet, in general, the whole-person approach to pain management takes into account that foods affect your body and mind, at times very noticeably. Although it's helpful to know what foods may help or hinder with regard to your particular health problem, what tends to be a trigger for most people may not be a trigger for you and vice versa.

Investing time in becoming your own detective with regard to what works for you will be worth the effort. You can enlist your doctor's help to this end. He may have valuable information to relay with regard to dietary recommendations based on your diagnoses and general health. If you have not yet had this discussion with your doctor, it is certainly worth asking what he generally advises, what the science says regarding your condition, and what he has observed other patients to benefit from. Although this type of advice does not represent "hard data" from randomized clinical trials, your doctor has the advantage of observing the impact of dietary changes on people who have something significant in common with you.

Diet and Mood

Despite the variable data with regard to diet and pain, it is known that pain and mood are strongly linked due to the many brain structures involved in both pain processing and emotion. There is research showing a nutrient-dense diet high in omega-3 fatty acids from fatty fish, walnuts, flaxseed, and the like, and that provides adequate zinc, B-vitamins, and magnesium should support a healthy mood. Certain B-vitamins, such as folate (otherwise known as vitamin B_9, or in fortified foods, folic acid) are essential for making neurotransmitters, the brain chemicals that very directly impact mood and pain. Conversely, deficiencies are associated with increased risk of depression, anxiety, sleep problems, and other physical symptoms. Thus, a diet that is balanced and supports a healthy mood and body can improve one's ability to function in general and cope with pain specifically.

Food vs. Dietary Supplements: What Is Best?

There is data specifically showing an effect of omega-3 fatty acid consumption and improvements in symptoms of rheumatoid arthritis. The findings are less consistent with regard to irritable bowel syndrome and asthma. Yet omega-3s are thought to decrease inflammation in general and support good overall health. Although there are some risks associated with the high levels of omega-3s found in supplements, such as decreased blood clotting (a problem for those taking blood thinners), these risks are not present when eating omega-3 rich foods. Foods high in omega-3s are fatty fish (e.g., salmon, mackerel, tuna), flaxseed and flaxseed oil, and walnuts.

FACT

In early 2015, the Dietary Guidelines Advisory Committee recommended that Americans consume water when thirsty, limit sugar and refined grains, and favor unsaturated fats, such as those found in fish, nuts, olive and vegetables oils, over saturated fats. For more diet tips, visit *http://healthfinder.gov*.

In general, the amount of any particular nutrient will be considerably lower when obtained through food versus supplements. Although this means you will be unable to consume extremely high levels of any particular nutrient through food alone, you will also gain the many other potentially beneficial aspects associated with foods (e.g., fiber, water content, phytochemicals, and other nutrients) that you will not get in the same way from taking a pill. And again, the safety of eating fresh, unprocessed foods is considerably greater than that of taking large doses of vitamins or other dietary supplements. Not to mention there is greater pleasure in eating a tasty, aromatic meal consisting of fresh, healthy food, ideally lovingly prepared by you or by someone you love (or at least by someone who is a good cook). In general, it's recommended that you speak with your doctor about your particular health issues, and what the general and specific recommendations are for you with regard to supplements and diet.

Food, Weight, Emotions, and Body Image

The relationship with food can be a complex one. So often, in addition to being how to fuel the body, food is used as a way to stuff down or distract from distressing thoughts or feelings. Meals can also have emotional associations that lead to over- or under-eating, such as positive memories of holiday celebrations, as well as recalling uncomfortable dinner-time conversations if your family dynamics were stressful. If eating feels like it offers comfort, or a welcome distraction, you may reach for food when you are tired, worried, lonely, angry, or in pain. If you are like a number of patients struggling with chronic pain and the myriad challenges that come with it, you may also feel like eating something sweet, fried, or salty is a "reward" for enduring difficulty.

Conversely, you may avoid food for these same reasons, as well as if you fear becoming overweight, experience a strong desire to "control" your body or your life, or use under-eating to rebel against others who are concerned about your weight.

In general, it's also easy to eat on automatic pilot and to make food choices that are convenient and calorie-dense but not particularly nutritious. In the industrialized world, food, for the most part, is plentiful. If you are like most people, there are probably many times when you miss a meal because you are busy or distracted and aren't particularly concerned about when you will be able to eat next—convenience and other foods are on every corner, so to speak. You may find yourself eating whatever is handy as part of the moment's multitasking—while surfing the Internet or responding to e-mails, watching TV, being on the phone, or driving somewhere. In these instances, you will have eaten without actually having been "present" for the experience. And that can interfere with fully enjoying and appreciating your food at the time or feeling sufficiently satisfied. You might even forget that you have eaten at all, because your mind was elsewhere.

The drive for food is inborn; your body and mind *know* that you need food—the right kind, in the right amount, with adequate frequency—not only to survive but also to *thrive*. When you are busy or experiencing stress, you may find it especially challenging to make healthy choices—even without the added issue of chronic pain. The presence of pain and, likely, the mood issues, cognitive changes, and fatigue that so often accompany it, can make it even less likely that you will feel up to eating well, particularly if this will involve extra planning and effort to make sure good food is available.

The Importance of Maintaining a Healthy Weight

As you now know, eating well is even more important for those who have a chronic pain condition. Both chronic pain and also underlying psychological issues related to eating can lead to your weight being either too high or too low. Each condition is associated with its own set of problems and also can exacerbate pain and decrease pain coping. Eating too little or too infrequently results in decreases in blood sugar and, therefore, decreases in physical energy and ability to concentrate. In addition, when you consume too few calories, you increase the likelihood of feeling weak, becoming light-headed, triggering a headache if you are prone to them, and other experiencing issues. If you have had issues with under-eating and body image previously, it will be even more important to be aware of them as you strive to eat well to manage pain.

Jenny—Under-eating as a Method of "Control"

Jenny had been an ultra-fit, ultra-lean college athlete and was now a "super woman" in her early 30s—a mother of two, a "perfect" wife to a successful professional. She had also been a frequent participant in weekend half marathons until a foot injury during a race led to the development of a complex regional pain syndrome. The associated temperature changes; electrical, burning, shooting pain; and frequent swelling initially made it feel impossible to even put a sneaker on, let alone run. Ever the trooper, Jenny gritted her teeth through a demanding course of physical therapy, pushing herself through high-level pain in the hopes that she could return to her previous "normal."

After several months of physical therapy, Jenny was able to once again wear shoes without agonizing pain, but could no longer engage in the high-intensity training that she was used to. Her decreased activity resulted in a fifteen-pound weight gain. "I can't believe I'm this heavy! No one looking at me now would believe that I did a triathlon—three times." Although Jenny's weight was still in the normal range, and she had been considered technically underweight previously, the changes in her body threatened her identity as a high-achieving person and athlete who had achieved a degree of mastery over her body. She found herself aware of significant fears of being "fat."

For the first time in her life, Jenny began seriously restricting her food intake in an effort to return to her pre-injury weight and body. After two months of skipping meals and decreasing her total calories, Jenny lost the fifteen pounds, but also complained of increased tearfulness, the onset of headaches, and decreased ability to cope with her pain. She had lost the weight she'd gained since her injury, but did not feel any better physically or emotionally. Addressing her fears in therapy and meeting with a registered dietitian helped her develop healthier eating habits and a more loving self-image over time. Although these efforts toward living more healthfully led to some weight gain, Jenny's mood and pain improved enough for her to become more functional and enjoy her life more.

The Problem of Overweight

Eating either too much food or too much processed, high calorie, nutrient-poor foods can cause weight gain in part due to unstable blood sugar (first too high and then too low), resulting in a vicious cycle of eating to compensate for swings in hunger and energy levels. Consuming processed foods can also increase feelings of fatigue and make your mood unstable. This is also attributable to the rapid changes in blood sugar and lack of nutrients associated with processed foods.

FACT

Many people who say their pain and fatigue prevent them exercising would adamantly refuse to carry twenty pounds of groceries around all day or lug an actual car tire around with them. But walking around with just twenty-two pounds of extra weight—the equivalent of the average car tire(!)—is also exhausting and can strain your back, joints, and patience.

In addition to exacerbating mood issues and feeling fatigued, weighing too much can put extra stress on already tender muscles and joints, worsen your gait, and further discourage you from moving your body.

Annie—Using Food as Comfort

Annie had struggled with multiple pain conditions for years, and by the time she was in her 30s she had seen seven different pain specialists and tried a number of medications, trigger point injections, and physical therapy. Although Annie noticed some temporary relief, she frequently reported significant sadness, fear, and resentment related to having to deal with pain at all, and with regard to her providers' collective inability to "cure" her of pain. She also felt her family was not sufficiently supportive of her. Annie longed for her parents and siblings to acknowledge how hard she struggled, and to offer to be more helpful, but she had a very difficult time communicating her needs directly.

Annie's one comfort was eating sweet, starchy food, and over the years her weight had increased to 290 pounds. Because the extra weight put a lot of pressure on her joints, Annie found physical therapy too painful and stopped going regularly. But this decision led her to feel depressed and angry with herself. When Annie's therapist attempted to discuss her use of food as a multipurpose tool—one for pushing away unpleasant emotions and distracting her from a body in pain—she burst into tears. "Sometimes I think that these treats are the *only things* that are always there for me—how can you talk about taking them away?" Annie sobbed forcefully as she disclosed this. "Besides, I've tried to lose weight before and it's never worked for me."

Because eating sweets made Annie feel better in the short term, she thought of this tool as one that helped her cope—a way of taking care of herself. If food remained Annie's main (or only) coping tool, it would continue to feel impossible for her to make changes in her diet and exercise that could improve her pain and give her a greater sense of control over her symptoms. It would also doom any diet program to ultimate failure—because part of her wanted to lose the weight, but another part felt this would be depriving her of something she needed. By this time, Annie knew a lot about what healthy eating should look like, so the work needed was to focus on helping her better understand the various meanings food had for her and develop other tools for dealing with stress.

The Healthy Pain-Management Diet

Two broad principles apply to eating well: Eat enough of healthy foods and consume sufficient water to remain adequately nourished and hydrated, and limit or avoid foods or substances that are nutrient-poor, worsen sleep, fatigue, or mood, or contribute to excess weight. Specifically, sugary, processed foods are more likely to make you feel worse shortly after eating them. Caffeine will wake you up initially but can contribute to irritability, insomnia, and may increase headaches or stomach upset in people who are vulnerable to those symptoms.

For most people, eating three solid meals or six mini meals will result in the greatest stability with regard to pain, mood, and blood sugar. Ideally, meals should be nutrient-dense, meaning they should consist of foods that together provide adequate amounts of protein, fats, carbohydrates, and fiber. They should also supply the necessary vitamins and minerals for good overall health.

Some tips for eating well:

- Select the least processed foods available (i.e., whole fruit instead of fruit juice, brown rice instead of white rice, a piece of broiled chicken instead of packaged chicken fingers)
- Strive to eat a variety of healthy foods in order to maximize your access to naturally occurring vitamins and minerals
- Limit or avoid alcohol consumption—especially if you are taking medications for mood, pain, or both
- Limit or avoid caffeine, particularly if you have difficulty sleeping
- Consume fiber-rich, natural foods (vegetables, fruits, whole grains, nuts) to ensure proper elimination and bowel function
- Drink plenty of water to remain hydrated
- Chew your food well, and make mealtime sacred—turn off the TV, get away from the computer, and really be present for the gift of the food in front of you

For more information on healthy eating in general, strategies for eating if you have a specific medical condition, as well as tips for eating when the goal is weight loss or weight gain, visit the website of the Academy of Nutrition and Dietetics: *www.eatright.org*.

When to Consult a Health Professional

Sometimes simply becoming more aware of unhealthy patterns and the specific changes you want to make can be enough to help you make necessary changes. Many of the tools mentioned in this book—movement therapies, guided imagery and hypnosis, and increasing your knowledge of healthy eating practices—can all help you in your efforts to feel better physically and emotionally and thus create positive change. If one of the following applies to you, however, it is strongly recommended that you consult with a health professional to discuss your issues with eating or body image:

WHEN TO SEEK HELP

- If your issues with eating, weight, or body image are long-standing
- If your issues with weight, eating, or body image have begun or worsened since your chronic pain developed
- If you have previously been diagnosed with an eating disorder and now are noticing a re-emergence of symptoms
- If you are pregnant or nursing and find yourself preoccupied with body image concerns
- If you are pregnant or nursing and feel significant fatigue or have difficulty planning a healthy diet
- If your weight or medical condition has led to other health problems, including fatigue, changes in heart rate, blood pressure, or cholesterol, or decreased ability to exercise
- If your weight or eating habits have led to increased pain frequency or severity
- If you have noticed feeling preoccupied with, or distressed about, your weight
- If a part of you wants to change your eating but feels unable to
- If you use eating to stifle emotions, distract from unpleasant thoughts, or "make up" for having experienced life difficulties (including pain)
- If friends, family, or your healthcare provider has expressed concern about your weight or eating habits
- If you desire more support with managing your weight, emotions, or both

A registered dietitian nutritionist, who will have an "RDN" as part of her credentials, is trained to help you come up with a specific plan for making dietary changes and achieve a healthy weight for your age, height, frame, and activity level.

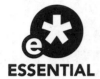

ESSENTIAL

The terms "nutritionist" and "dietitian" are often used interchangeably, but they are not equivalent. Many people may call themselves "nutritionists" but have little or even no formal education in nutrition. An RDN will have achieved at least a bachelor's degree in nutrition, as well as supervised practice hours, and passed a national exam. For more information on the credentialing of RDNs, visit: *www.eatright.org/resource/food/*.

A licensed psychotherapist, such as a psychologist, clinical social worker, or licensed mental health counselor, can help you understand your particular barriers to eating well, address any issues with self-esteem or body image, and work with you to create a step-by-step plan for healthy change. You can find a psychotherapist who is both licensed and experienced in working with chronic pain and weight or eating issues by contacting your state's licensing boards or psychological association, or via reputable online directories of mental health professionals. The two most well known are *www.psychologytoday.com* and *www.goodtherapy.org*.

Tools and Apps for Tracking Your Diet

An old staple of food monitoring is the three-day diary. This involves writing down everything you eat and drink, and in the amounts consumed, for a three-day period. Food diaries are helpful for a number of reasons. First, keeping one will help you become more aware of what you tend to eat and drink, in what amounts, and when. For example, if you tend to drink an extra cup of coffee and reach for a candy bar around 3 P.M. on the days you chart, this can tell you about how your energy probably fluctuates during the day and help you look for other solutions.

Second, if you have weight issues (either too high or too low), it can help you get a more accurate understanding of how many calories you tend to consume and whether you need to make changes with regard to what you are eating, how much, or how often. Record the time of day, what you ate and drank, and how much you consumed of each item. You can do this simply and inexpensively by getting an old-fashioned paper notebook for this purpose so you don't feel constrained with regard to how much you write. Just include the following headings:

SAMPLE FOOD DIARY ENTRIES

Time	Foods and Beverages	Comments
7:00 A.M.	12 oz. coffee with 2 tablespoons half-and-half	Feeling sleepy and craving another cup
8:30 A.M.	2 fried eggs on a plain bagel, with 1 tablespoon cream cheese	Really hungry today
9:30 A.M.	1 granola bar	Can't believe I'm hungry again already, feeling tired
3:00 P.M.	2 slices of plain pizza, 1 (12-ounce) can diet soda	Ate late lunch, really hungry, developed headache at 11 A.M. and didn't subside until after I ate lunch
6:00 P.M.	16 ounces coffee with 3 tablespoons half-and-half, large apple	Had coffee and snack while driving home
7:00 P.M.	large salad with 3 cups of romaine, 4 ounces grilled chicken, chopped carrots and celery, and 4 tablespoons of ranch dressing; large glass of water	Aiming to have healthier food to make up for the rest of the day's choices. Still hungry after dinner
8:30 P.M.	½ cup lite vanilla ice cream with ¼ cup frozen blueberries	Dessert while watching TV
12:30 A.M.	10 crackers with peanut butter	Couldn't sleep—too jittery. Craved comfort food.

If you are unsure about how to estimate the amount you have consumed, it's worth investing in some measuring cups and spoons. In the comments section, you can note anything else that seems relevant.

There's an App for That

If you prefer to go the more high-tech route, there are a number of smartphone apps that can help you record your food intake and even look up the nutrient facts of processed foods. Here are a few popular ones in no particular order:

- MyNetDiary is a free app for iOS and Android that lets you track food servings, calories, and nutrients, helps with meal planning, and includes a barcode scanner for scanning prepared foods for the nutrient data. It also allows you to track your exercise, read information logged on other fitness apps, and get support from an online community. Visit *www .mynetdiary.com*.

- Calorie Counter and Diet Tracker by MyFitnessPal is a free app for iOS and Android that allows you to track calories, nutrients, and exercise, use a barcode scanner for packaged food, and connect with an online community. In addition, the app allows you to connect with over fifty devices and other apps to help you achieve your goals. It also features a recipe importer that lets you view any recipe on the web and import and track it with the app. Visit *www.myfitnesspal.com*.
- Diet and Food Tracker by SparkPeople is a free app for iOS and Android. It has a food tracking database with over 3 million foods, a barcode scanner, a daily weigh-in page, GPS tracking to let you know how far you've walked or jogged, exercise demos, and more. For this and other related apps by this company, including a Healthy Recipe app, visit *www.sparkpeople.com/mobile-apps.asp*.

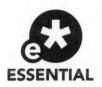

ESSENTIAL

Remember not to get too caught up in looking up foods and calorie counts; the main goal is that you gain insight into what you're eating and why, and get feedback when you make healthy changes. Feedback reinforces positive choices and helps you stick with them.

Food, Pain, and Mood Tracking

Another very valuable tool is to chart your food intake and also note your mind and body symptoms (e.g., pain, mood, digestive issues or headaches, etc.) before and after you eat. What you learn may seem simple, but it can be a very, very powerful tool in terms of how you manage your health and well-being. For example, Joe found that his irritability and headaches increased if he waited more than half an hour after waking up to eat breakfast. Leslie realized that having rice and gluten-free grain products seemed soothing to her irritable bowel syndrome (IBS), but eating anything containing wheat increased cramping and diarrhea. And Mitchell found that he could have one cup of coffee in the morning without much impact on his body, but any more than that and his sleep would be disrupted and fibromyalgia pain increased.

Charting your intake of foods that you suspect may improve or worsen your symptoms and the impact each food has on your body can give you more power to decide how you will feel on a given day. To track, simply add this information in the comments section, create a symptom-specific column, or create columns for both physical symptoms and changes in mood. So, your diary headings could be:

Time	Food and Beverage	Mood (before and after)	Pain (before and after)	Comments

You can even eliminate a particular food for a week and chart any difference you notice when reintroducing it to your diet. Are your symptoms worse? Better? No different? Of course, there are now apps that can help you keep track of not only your food intake but also pain or other symptoms, all in the same place. Some apps will allow you to print out a PDF summary to bring to your doctor or dietitian.

Imagery to Help with Dietary Changes

As you already know, and you will learn more about in other chapters, your mind exerts a powerful influence on how you feel physically and emotionally, on what you believe is possible for you, and with regard to the behaviors you change effectively. Self-hypnosis and guided imagery can help you more easily let go of the old ways of doing things and make healthier changes. The following is some imagery you can record in your own voice or ask someone else to record for you. Listen daily or as often as you like to help you more easily make healthy, self-loving food choices. The ellipses (. . .) indicate places where you should pause before reading the next phrase. When listening, you may wish to get a glass of water to keep nearby so you can take a few sips to help re-orient you afterward.

Hypnotic Imagery for Eating Well

Take a few moments that are just for you . . . allowing your body to find the most comfortable position for you . . . whatever that is, right now. And it doesn't need to be anything in particular . . . there is no such thing as perfect . . . and that's a wonderful thing . . . and you can simply observe your breath for the moment . . . just noticing the natural exhalation . . . and inhalation . . . with each cycle of breath allowing yourself to become even more comfortable . . . just like that. . . . And in your mind's eye, notice the healthy changes that the healthiest part of you desires to make . . . allowing yourself to choose foods that are nourishing . . . and healing . . . that help your body and mind feel balanced . . . and clear . . . with good energy . . . and enhanced comfort . . . your wisest self knows exactly what these will be . . . fresh fruits . . . and vegetables . . . their colors bright . . . and vibrant . . . taking in their scent . . . lean proteins . . . in just the right amount . . . and complex carbohydrates . . . everything in the most natural state . . . seasoned lovingly . . . to bring out their flavors . . . healthy fats to keep your mind balanced and help you feel satisfied . . . your body's wisdom knows exactly what's best for you, the you you are now . . . and the you you are creating . . . the appeal of clear, fresh water growing every day . . . hydrating your cells . . . balancing your energy . . . as you take care of yourself in the most loving way possible . . . making healthy choices . . . in just the right amount . . . fueling your body . . . giving it what is healthy . . . because over time, our tastes very naturally change . . . developing a more sophisticated palate . . . and if any part of you worries about making change . . . that's perfectly fine . . . it's completely normal to feel some adjustment when you realize that the ways that worked before are different from what you need now . . . because now you know better, and so you can do well . . . and feel wonderful . . . allowing some of the choices of the past to remain there . . . with gratitude for whatever they did then . . . so you can move forward . . . so much wiser . . . so much easier now . . . to make healthy choices . . . the most loving thing . . . and be well . . . wonderful. . . .

So, just allow yourself to trust yourself . . . the part of you that is always looking out for you . . . partnering with you to help you feel your best . . . and taking loving care of you. . . . And once again, bring your attention back to your breathing . . . so nice and relaxed . . . becoming more aware of the sounds in the room, your body in the present . . . feeling relaxed but fully awake, and with a few deep breaths, and some sips of water, you are ready to return to your day.

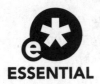

ESSENTIAL

If you are new to imagery or hypnosis, and are unfamiliar with the slower-than-normal pacing, you may wish to listen to a free audio sample before recording a track for yourself. Here is a link to a hypnosis track for achieving a healthy weight and body image: *www.healthjourneys.com/ Store/Products/Healthy-Weight-Body-Image/716.*

CHAPTER 7

Exercise and Movement Therapies

Your body is your most steadfast companion and ally, even if you are in pain. When you are feeling emotionally overloaded, your body will strive to communicate this to you via symptoms that are "louder" or more intense. When you have either overdone activity or been too sedentary, your body will let you know this as well. Getting the right amount and type of exercise can help you regain lost function, work through any sadness, anxiety, or grief, and feel more confident and centered, despite pain.

The Effects of Prolonged Sitting

If you are like most people, other than professional dancers or athletes, you are probably unaware of your physical posture more often than not. And if you spend much of your time sitting, whether for work, leisure, or due to pain, your muscles may have become used to being in a contracted, pulled-forward posture. Sitting for most of the day, as millions of people do, is linked to disc problems, muscle atrophy, joint and muscle aches and stiffness, and poor circulation. All of these issues can worsen an existing pain condition and even create new ones. In addition, having weak abdominal muscles decreases core stability, making you more vulnerable to losing your balance (and thus, potential injury) when moving.

Of even greater concern than these issues is that prolonged sitting is associated with higher body fat (even if you workout otherwise), increased risk of cardiovascular disease, high blood sugar, and a 50 percent increase in mortality from any cause. In fact, watching even four hours of television per day has been found to increase the risk of health problems. Unfortunately, chances are, if you are in pain, you are moving less than you used to, and possibly not very much at all.

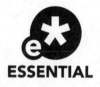

ESSENTIAL

Starting and sticking with an exercise program can feel daunting, especially if you have not been active in some time. Setting concrete, specific, and small goals will make it much easier to recognize progress and stick with your exercise plan. For example, if your goal is to walk for a half hour, you can begin by committing to walking for five minutes.

"May the Force Be with You"

You may have heard the phrases, "A body in motion tends to stay in motion" and "A body at rest tends to remain at rest." These paraphrase the "Law of Inertia," put forth by seventeenth-century mathematician and physicist Sir Isaac Newton. More specifically, this law states that in order for the movement (or not) of an object to change, an "external force" must act upon it.

You can observe this law "in action," so to speak, by throwing a baseball across a field. If not for the external force of gravity, pulling the ball toward the earth until it falls, the ball would forever continue on its path at the same speed. The Law of Inertia also states, in effect, that if you were to walk across that same field later and find the ball on the ground, it would remain in the same place until an external force—perhaps a strong wind, or someone picking it up and throwing it once again—caused it to move.

Even if you don't recall learning about Sir Isaac in your junior high science class, it's worth noting that the longer your own body remains at rest, the more challenging it will be (and the greater "force" it will require) to get moving again, albeit for different reasons than Sir Isaac referenced when he came up with the Law of Inertia. In fact, if you have ever tried to restart an exercise program after being sedentary for some time, you may have noticed that it required more energy or exertion on your part to, for example, walk or jog a mile than it used to. Relatedly, you may also have noticed that it has taken a greater degree of mental or emotional energy (an internal force) or perhaps nagging by your doctor or family members (external forces) to get you moving again.

FACT

Kinesiophobia is the fear of movement and re-injury, and can be quite common among those in pain. This fear can lead you to avoid activity that is actually essential to your regaining some physical and social functioning, improving mood, and reclaiming your life. Exposure therapy (a type of CBT treatment) and activity pacing can help you conquer your fear.

Pain, anxiety, depression, fatigue, nausea, and feelings of self-consciousness, grief, or resentment about the changes in your body can all act as internal forces working *against* change. In addition, any stereotypes you may have held without previously being aware of them can get in the way of your being active. For example, if you associate getting older with naturally becoming more sedentary, you think exercise is futile past a certain age, or you believe that pain means you need to rest and avoid exerting yourself, you will be much less likely to move. And yet, movement is essential to prevent your physical and emotional health from deteriorating over time. Even those without a chronic pain or other medical condition will develop increasing health problems and have decreased physical functioning if they don't move.

Human beings have a natural tendency to compare themselves to others, but comparing your fitness progress to someone else's (or your own, prior to having pain) is unfair to you and can derail your efforts to exercise. Unless comparisons motivate and inspire you, you are better off leaving them behind.

Exercise As a Key to Better Health

Even if you were not a very active person prior to developing pain, increasing your activity level now can help you enhance your health and well-being. Exercise has been associated with the following benefits:

- Improved immune functioning
- Increased heart health
- Improved blood sugar
- Improved digestion and decreased constipation
- Reduced risk of a number of cancers
- Better hormonal balance
- Increased hardiness in the face of life stresses
- Better, more restful sleep
- Improved mood and sense of well-being

Pacing is key when beginning an exercise regimen, as it reduces the risk of injury and overdoing it. You are most likely to remain motivated if you set small, specific, and achievable goals. If your goal is to walk two miles, and you currently can only walk one block, you might begin by walking one block every day for two weeks, adding another to your routine for the next week or two, and so on.

Exercise Helps (Literally!) Build a Better Brain

The prevailing thought in medicine used to be that once you entered adulthood, your brain could no longer develop or grow. In effect, many believed that your brain function might get worse over time, but certainly it would not get any better. One of the most exciting and surprising findings of the past few years is that exercise facilitates the creation of new neurons in the brain. This effect is the result of increased blood flow to the brain and new blood vessels forming from existing ones. In addition, exercise increases the amount of a specific protein in the brain called "brain-derived neurotrophic factor," or BDNF.

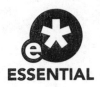

ESSENTIAL

Everyone experiences some ups and downs on the road to making significant change. Remember that setbacks and challenges are a normal part of the process, and try to keep the bigger picture in mind—that exercise will give you back some feeling of control over your body and make it easier to do many of the things you want to.

In essence, exercise is in and of itself a very powerful tool for improving health and well-being throughout your entire body—brain included.

Specific Brain Benefits

Scientists have discovered a number of ways that exercise benefits the brain beyond growing new neurons. Here are five of them:

1. Reduction in age-related cognitive decline—even in those carrying a gene for Alzheimer's
2. Improvements in cognitive ability—including working memory, reaction time, language skills, verbal learning, visual-spatial skills, reading and math skills, and executive functioning (the abilities to plan, pay attention, and make decisions based on logic)
3. Reduced severity of depression symptoms and, possibly, reduced risk of becoming depressed even in the face of stress
4. Improved sleep even in those who have anxiety or depression symptoms
5. Increased resistance to developing a panic attack

Exercise as "Medicine"

For many, the perceived mental and physical barriers to exercising can seem to outweigh the positives. And yet, if there were a single pill that could enhance mood and physical functioning, reduce disease risk, and cause the brain to sprout new neurons, every single doctor in America would prescribe it! Such a pill would go a long way to solving much of the world's health problems. The drug company to develop it would make billions, if not trillions, of dollars. And you might personally save thousands upon thousands of dollars in personal healthcare costs due to your improved health. Yet exercise in many forms is absolutely free. And if you think about exercise in this way, it may just inspire you to get moving.

Exercise for Pain Management

Exercise in general is thought to reduce pain severity and improve pain coping. Different types of exercise can improve your health and alleviate pain, albeit by different mechanisms.

Aerobic exercise, also referred to as "cardio," involves sustained movement that elevates your heart rate and rate of breathing. Examples of aerobic exercise include brisk walking, swimming, biking, jogging, and dancing, among others. Engaging in aerobic exercise probably reduces pain through the release of endorphins, your body's natural opiates. Engaging in regular aerobic exercise is also associated with reduced disability.

Strength training, also referred to as resistance training, involves challenging your skeletal muscles to fatigue, and then allowing at least a day in between these exercises for the muscles to rest and repair, becoming stronger and firmer over time. Another name for strength training is "resistance training," and the resistance can come in the form of lifting weights, using your own body (such as when you do a push up, abdominal crunch, lunge, or squat), or using resistance bands.

Developing strong muscles will improve your metabolism because even at rest, muscle tissue is more "metabolically active," meaning it burns more calories than fat tissue does. Strong muscles will also improve your ability to do the things you want and need to do, whether pick up a small child, carry groceries, or just get from one place to another. Furthermore, if your muscles are strong, you will be less likely to fall or otherwise injure or strain yourself when engaging in daily activities. Having strong muscles can help you change your self-concept from that of a person whose body is weak, fragile, or "dis-abled" to that of a strong, effective person who may also have health challenges. How you think of yourself is especially important because this will determine how confident you are and how likely you are to engage in life fully, despite pain.

FACT

Researchers at Harvard and the National Cancer Institute looked at data from over 600,000 people and found that non-exercisers had the highest risk of early death. Getting even a little bit of exercise lowered the risk by 20 percent. Doing 150 minutes of exercise a week (about 22 minutes per day) lowered the risk of premature death by 31 percent!

Stretching exercises improve flexibility and help keep your body balanced. They are also very helpful for reducing muscular tension and alleviating stress, and can help decrease pain severity. Ideally, stretching should be gentle, and stretches should be held for at least thirty seconds each to allow the muscle time to ease into lengthening. Stretching can be done on your own, at home, as part of an exercise class, or with assistance from your physical therapist. Yoga and Pilates are two types of exercises that incorporate lengthening and balancing of muscles into fluid series of motion.

Which Exercises Are Most Helpful?

As you might imagine, if your pain is related to problems with bones or joints, you will likely want to avoid exercises that are jarring, such as jogging. Low-impact exercises, like walking and swimming, should still provide benefits with regard to heart health, stress reduction, pain management, and overall well-being. Your particular medical condition and your doctor's advice will probably determine which specific exercises are considered most appropriate for you, and your program should be adapted as you become more fit. The general consensus is to strive to move on most days of the week, regardless of what type of exercise you choose.

Strength Training, Aerobic, or Stretching?

Ideally, your exercise program will keep you feeling strong, flexible, and help you have the endurance to do what you need to on a daily basis—whatever that means for you given your current health status. Therefore, your program should incorporate all three types of exercise to build strength, enhance stamina, and develop greater flexibility and range of motion around your joints. As you train your body over time, your body will adapt to the demands you have placed on it, and your exercises should seem easier to do. At this point, consult with your doctor or physical therapist about how to take your program to the next level.

With regard to the research on exercise types and pain relief, a recent review of forty-eight studies of exercise for those with knee osteoarthritis found that the greatest reductions in pain and disability were obtained by engaging in regular exercise—whether aerobic or strength training—at least three times per week. The researchers looking at these studies, which included data on over four thousand people, concluded that there was no difference in benefit between strength training and aerobic exercise programs, as long as they were structured, goal-oriented, performed at least three or more times weekly, and emphasized one broad type of exercise per session.

In studies of patients with fibromyalgia, aerobic exercise has been shown to improve symptoms of pain, fatigue, depression and increase health-related quality of life. Strength training has been linked to improved general well-being and physical functioning. Combining both strength training and aerobic exercise has been associated with improved physical functioning and reductions in pain. And aquatic exercises have been shown to improve all of this, as well as mood symptoms.

Tai Chi and Qigong

Tai chi and Qigong are practices that have existed for thousands of years, long before the emergence of Western ideas about exercise or healing. Both tai chi and Qigong fall under the heading of Traditional Chinese Medicine, or TCM, and share emphases on purposeful, fluid movement, focused attention, and breathing.

These practices originated thousands of years ago as Chinese martial arts. Tai chi is characterized by controlled breathing and slow, graceful movements that are said to mimic the movements of animals. Tai chi practice enhances flexibility, improves feelings of well-being, decreases stress, and is thought to balance "chi" or "qi," also known as "life force energy."

Qigong, sometimes referred to as Qi Gong, also is purported to move and balance one's own chi. Although in the Western world you will probably hear Qigong described as a single type of practice, there are reportedly thousands of forms of Qigong, some developed as a spiritual practice, some for medical or health-related purposes, and others as martial arts.

Like tai chi, Qigong is characterized by flowing movements, is believed to enhance health via balancing qi, and fosters a sense of relaxation and peace. During *internal* Qigong, the person practicing it balances his own energy via the movements, breathing, and focused attention. *External* Qigong involves a trained practitioner diagnosing and balancing the qi of another person.

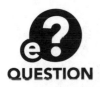

QUESTION

What is the "best" exercise?
The "best" type of exercise, as stated beautifully by Dr. Christiane Northrup, is "the one you will do." If you have been sedentary due to pain, your first and most important exercise goal may be to commit to moving on most days of the week. Discuss with your doctor what the most appropriate program is for you. You can increase the intensity and duration as your body gets more used to moving.

Tai Chi, Qigong, and Health

Although studies of tai chi to date have been small, the research thus far supports what many practitioners report with regard to tai chi's benefits. Specifically, tai chi has been linked to improved balance and reduced risk of falls, enhanced feelings of well-being, better cardiovascular fitness, improved blood pressure, and enhanced immune function in those who have had shingles.

A recent study funded in part by NCCIH found that one-hour sessions of tai chi practiced in a twice-weekly class for twelve weeks, plus at-home practice, and then practiced solely at home for another twelve weeks resulted in improved sleep, mood, and quality of life in patients with fibromyalgia. The researchers found that the improvements were still maintained six months later. Other studies have found that tai chi reduced musculoskeletal pain, depression, and improved quality of life.

FACT

The NCCIH has a five-part video series, totaling about fifteen minutes, discussing tai chi and Qigong, as well as their health benefits. The videos also demonstrate the flowing poses and breathing characteristic of these practices. To view the videos, visit *https://nccih.nih.gov/video/taichidvd-full.*

Another large-scale review of the research looked at results from seventy-seven studies involving either tai chi or internal Qigong practice. Over six thousand participants were enrolled in these trials. Because of what the authors of this review described as innate similarities between the approaches, and because both Qigong and tai chi movements tend to be simplified when used as a research intervention, they were considered equivalent practices for the purpose of this analysis.

The review concluded that tai chi and Qigong practice were associated with significant improvements in bone health, cardiopulmonary fitness, physical function, falls prevention and balance, general quality of life, immunity, and reduced anxiety and depression. In addition, Qigong and tai chi practice were linked to greater feelings of self-efficacy (the belief you can do what you need to do). Self-efficacy is important because you are more likely to make positive changes for yourself if you believe you can.

Yoga

Yoga is at once a meditative practice, physical discipline, and philosophy. Yoga originated in ancient India as part of Ayurveda, the Indian traditional medical system. There are several different forms of yoga that have become popular in the West. According to the 2007 National Health Interview Survey conducted by the National Institutes of Health, yoga is the sixth most commonly used complementary health practice among adults, with an estimated 16 million adults practicing in the United States. The survey also found that more than 1.5 million children practiced yoga in the previous year.

Like tai chi and Qigong, yoga is characterized by focused attention, flowing movements, specific postures (called *asanas*), and controlled use of the breath (*pranayama*). The practice of yoga can enhance flexibility, improve stability, help relieve tension in tight tissues, strengthen muscles, and improve endurance. Furthermore, taking yoga classes can reduce social isolation. Those who practice regularly often report feelings of improved peace, well-being, and resistance to stress.

The Yoga Research

The NCCIH describes the research on yoga in more detail, but to summarize, studies of yoga for chronic lower back pain have found that practicing yoga was linked to reductions in pain, disability, and depression. The mechanisms by which yoga helps are unclear, but it has been suggested that yoga may lead to the release of endorphins, reduction of inflammation, or enhanced blood flow. A 2011 review of ten studies involving a total of nearly 500 participants found that yoga helped reduce pain related to osteoarthritis, labor, migraines, carpal tunnel, and lower back pain. The authors cautioned that more research needs to be done to reach a definitive conclusion about yoga as a pain management tool, but the results are promising.

Other research has shown yoga to likely have benefits with regard to smoking cessation, reducing fatigue in breast cancer survivors, promoting a healthy weight in general, and weight loss in those needing to lose weight. A recent study found that regular yoga practice was linked to improved pain tolerance as compared to those who did not practice yoga. Furthermore, experienced yoga practitioners had increased gray matter volume in brain regions associated with pain processing, pain regulation, and attention. This finding is not surprising, given the emphasis on mindfully observing discomfort without attaching to, judging, or otherwise reacting to it. For more information about the research on yoga and health, and to view an informative video about some of the findings described here, visit *https://nccih.nih.gov/video/yoga*.

There's an App for That

As you might imagine, there are a number of apps available to help you get motivated to get moving and keep up your exercise regimen. Many are free or low cost, and some will also enable you to track your food and calorie intake. The latter will be helpful if you need to lose or gain weight as part of your plan to improve overall health and reduce pain. The app you choose may also depend on what exercise plan is most appropriate for you at present given your current health and fitness status:

- FitStar is an app that aims to provide the personalized feedback one would normally only receive from a personal trainer. The workouts are customizable based on parameters you set, including your current level of fitness and the goals you set for yourself. As you become more fit, the app increases the difficulty of the workouts. The app is available in both a general version: *http://fitstar.com/#top*, and a yoga one: *https://itunes.apple.com/us/app/fitstar-yoga/*. The basic versions of each are free, and there are options for paid upgrades. For use with the iPhone, iPad, and Apple TV.
- Map My Run is an app whose name fails to reflect the over 600 activities the app is purported to be able to track with regard to time, distance, level of intensity, and calories burned. The app features a GPS that allows you to track your journey on a virtual map during your walk, run, or bike ride. You can also track your calorie intake. The app is compatible with several activity tracking devices, including the Jawbone, Misfit, and Fitbit. It's available for free on the iPhone and iPod Touch, and there is also a paid version with additional features. Access it here: *https://itunes.apple.com*.
- The *New York Times* 7-minute workout is based on data showing you can increase your fitness by doing a series of simple exercises for a mere seven minutes each day. The exercises use your own body weight as the resistance, and part of the benefit comes from moving from one exercise to the next without a rest in between. Exercising in this way keeps your heart rate elevated and can help you get fit with minimal investment in time. Because of the high level of intensity, it's probably only appropriate for those who are somewhat fit to begin with. *http://well.blogs.nytimes.com/projects/workouts/*

- The WebMD-Trusted Health and Wellness Information App, designed for use with the iPhone and iPod Touch, is among the most comprehensive wellness apps out there. It is free and allows you to connect an activity tracker, wireless scale, or blood pressure monitor. It also features a symptom checker, healthy lifestyle tips, and more. Access it here: *https:// itunes.apple.com/app/id295076329.*

Activity Trackers

The apps here do not require activity trackers, but if you like the idea of having a wearable device that gives you direct feedback about your daily activity and also can sync with your phone as well as more high-tech apps, you may want to look into purchasing an exercise tracker. The pros of an exercise tracker are that for many people, it provides that extra bit of feedback that motivates them to keep moving.

For example, if your goal is to take ten thousand steps per day (a total of about five miles daily), and you notice you are one thousand steps short of the day's goal, feedback from a device may be what prompts you to take the stairs, walk somewhere rather than driving (if this is feasible), or delay watching TV until your activity goal is met. Several of the trackers also monitor sleep duration and quality. Trackers tend to cost somewhere between $100 and $200. Here are brief overviews of just a few of the more popular ones:

- The Jawbone Up 24 is a device that tracks your active time and steps taken as well as inactive time. It features an inactivity alert that can let you know when you have been sedentary for too long and encourage you to move around. The device also tracks your sleep duration and quality, and features an alarm that will vibrate ahead of your wakeup time to help you feel more refreshed (and is less jarring than a conventional alarm). Jawbone recently released an app that lets you track your caffeine intake. The Jawbone works with both iOS and Android devices. For more information, visit *www.jawbone.com.*
- The Fitbit Flex is comparatively tiny and can be worn on a rubber bracelet or placed in a pocket. A unique feature is that it is water-resistant (not waterproof). The Fitbit vibrates and lights up when you meet your

exercise goals. It also tracks distance and calories as well as sleep length and depth. For more information, visit *www.fitbit.com/flex*.

- The Misfit Shine is tiny and easily hidden for those who do not wish to show off their exercise trackers. The device attaches to most items of clothing via a very strong magnet, but can also be worn on the wrist via a rubber watchband. The Shine is powered by a watch battery, so it won't need recharging, as other trackers do. It's also waterproof so it can be worn while swimming. Finally, the Shine tracks duration and quality of sleep. It's compatible with both iOS and Android devices. For more information, visit *www.misfitwearables.com*.

Your "Stance" Can Change Your Life

In 2010, Columbia University researchers Dana Carney and Andy Yap and Harvard Business School professor Amy Cuddy published simple but impactful findings about how changing your posture could significantly improve your body chemistry and enhance your confidence. In fact, doing so for a mere two minutes led to a measurable decrease in cortisol (a stress hormone) and an increase in testosterone (a hormone that increases feelings of confidence). Furthermore, the team found that two minutes of "power posing" shifted participants' perspectives with regard to risk; they became more likely to see "risk" as an opportunity for success, rather than an opportunity for failure.

The team described power posing as adopting a stance that is expansive—arms and legs wide, such as the "Wonder Woman" pose— legs hip-width apart, hands on hips, chin and gaze level. Similarly, standing with legs grounded and apart, and hands reaching toward the sky, or sitting reclined with legs out straight and arms behind the head also led to positive mind-body changes.

You may wonder what prompted the researchers to even consider the question: Can your posture change your body and mind? The team was already aware that confident people tend to take up more physical space (via expansive postures) and have higher levels of testosterone and lower levels of cortisol. Conversely, people who feel less confident tend to adopt contractive, protective postures (think of sitting with your arms and legs crossed, slightly hunched forward), have higher levels of cortisol, and lower testosterone.

Why Posture Is Important in Pain Management

All the aspects common to the pain experience, including depression, anxiety, hopelessness, and helplessness, as well as grief related to bodily and life changes, tend to reinforce poor self-image, fear of making change, and even anger at your body. None of these outcomes is helpful. You may very well feel overwhelmed by the thought of starting an exercise program, but you can probably commit to two minutes of practicing just about anything. Changing your posture could be the first step to reclaiming your body and your sense of yourself as an effective and *powerful* agent of change.

FACT

In Professor Cuddy's Ted Talk, "Your Body Language Shapes Who You Are," she discusses the power-posing research as well as surviving an accident that left her with brain damage and unable to walk. She later made a remarkable recovery, returned to school, and went on to become Harvard faculty. Her inspiring talk has been viewed nearly 25 million times as of this writing. To view her talk, visit *www.youtube.com/watch?v=Ks-_Mh1QhMc*.

CHAPTER 8

Dietary Supplements

Americans spend upwards of $20 billion annually on dietary supplements. These include vitamins, minerals, herbal preparations, and sports-related supplements. When making decisions related to dietary supplements, it's important first to know what the officially recommended amounts are for specific vitamins and minerals. Here is a link to the National Institutes of Health, Office of Dietary Supplements page on nutrient recommendations: *http://ods.od.nih.gov*. This resource should serve as a helpful general guideline.

Supplements Overview

If you have chronic pain, you probably wonder which supplements may be additionally helpful, in what amounts, and for which symptoms or conditions. The answers to these questions are not always clear-cut, for a few reasons. First, different supplements have varying amounts of research-derived evidence suggesting they are helpful for a specific condition. Second, there may be limited information as to how certain supplements interact with other supplements, foods, or prescribed medications. Third, there may be limited information about how safe a particular supplement is. Further complicating the issue, because supplements are poorly regulated in the United States, the quality of a particular supplement can vary significantly from brand to brand.

ALERT

Herbal and vitamin supplements run the gamut with regard to consistency of ingredients and may contain contaminants. Consumerlab.com is an independent laboratory that evaluates supplements and provides detailed reviews of the research. You can also look for products that have been vetted by the United States Pharmacopeial Convention (*www.usp.org*) or NSF International, which develops public health standards: *www.nsf.org*.

Anxiety and depression are commonly associated with chronic pain. Many of the supplements described here have benefits beyond those outlined in the following section. Additionally, there may be other supplements not featured here that are also helpful and appropriate for your particular condition. Note that what you will find here is not encyclopedic, but the supplements included in this chapter have some evidence of benefit for at least one pain or mood issue, are considered low risk, and several generally contribute to good overall health. The doses listed are based on the research to date, but as the research is continually evolving, the recommendations are not clear-cut. Be proactive in learning about updates to the findings and recommendations about particular supplements. You can access this information in easy-to-understand language by visiting the NIH's Office of Dietary Supplements at *http://ods.od.nih.gov*.

ALERT

Since some supplements may not be right for you, or may need to be taken at a different dose than what is generally recommended, discuss any supplements you are considering taking with your doctor. She can advise you of potential side effects, interactions with medications, and when you should avoid a particular supplement completely.

SAMe

S-adenosyl-methionine (SAMe) is a compound that occurs naturally in the body. SAMe is found in every cell, and plays a role in the manufacture of important brain chemicals, such as serotonin and dopamine. SAMe is also involved in the formation of cartilage. Normally, your body will make all the SAMe it needs; however, if you are deficient in the amino acid methionine, or the vitamins folate and B_{12}, you may become deficient in SAMe.

The strongest research findings to date have found that supplementing with SAMe can help reduce pain, stiffness, and inflammation due to osteoarthritis as effectively as some prescribed medications. Keep in mind that it will take longer for you to notice a pain reduction benefit from SAMe than it will from anti-inflammatory drugs.

There is also moderate-level evidence that SAMe is effective for treating mild-to-moderate depression. In some studies, SAMe was as effective as antidepressant medications, and it tends to work more quickly. The addition of SAMe to an antidepressant regimen has also been shown to help improve depression symptoms in people who have not responded well to antidepressants alone.

Although there is less evidence supporting the use of SAMe for fibromyalgia, and other, non-pain related conditions, both some research and anecdotal evidence support using SAMe for improved energy, concentration, and decreased pain in general.

What You Should Know

SAMe appears to be safe for most people, with the most common side effect being mild, transient digestive upset. This can be minimized by beginning with small doses of SAMe and increasing to therapeutic levels gradually.

Because SAMe is involved in neurotransmitter (brain chemical) production, you should consult your doctor before adding it to your regimen. Relatedly, you should avoid taking SAMe if you have bipolar disorder, as well as if you are already taking antidepressants or other medications that influence your brain's chemistry, unless your doctor gives you clearance to take this supplement *and* is willing to monitor you. The reason for caution here is to avoid triggering a manic episode; developing a serotonin syndrome, which can be harmful and possibly fatal; or having an adverse supplement-drug interaction.

Therapeutic doses of SAMe are described as about 400 mg three times daily on an empty stomach. You may notice a benefit at a lower dose, however, perhaps even as low as 200 mg once daily if your weight is low or if you are especially sensitive to medications or supplements. A good general rule is to "start low and go slow"—increasing only to what you need to feel a therapeutic effect.

It's important to take adequate folate with SAMe to avoid an unhealthy elevation in homocysteine levels (this is especially important for patients with cardiovascular issues). Taking 400 mcg of l-methylfolate, the form of supplemental folate most easily used by the body, is usually sufficient; however, if you have a genetic mutation known as MTHFR, you may require a higher dose of l-methylfolate or another folate supplement that your doctor feels is appropriate for you.

Finally, SAMe is a relatively expensive supplement that is not covered by insurance. It's worth considering whether the monthly expense of a therapeutic dose is feasible for you.

Vitamin D

There has been a lot of talk about vitamin D lately, and with good reason. Low levels of vitamin D are associated with increased risk of rheumatoid arthritis, muscle and bone weakness, cardiovascular disease, uterine fibroids, and depression. There are two forms of the vitamin that you have likely heard about—D_2 and D_3. D_3 is the form that is made from exposure to sunlight and can also be obtained by eating fatty fish such as sardines and mackerel, beef liver, egg yolks, and fortified milk, among other foods.

Vitamin D, taken with calcium, is associated with decreased risk of bone loss and bone fractures in menopausal women, and in general, vitamin D is essential for good bone health. Several studies have shown that vitamin D supplementation is associated with better muscle strength and balance in older adults, may reduce inflammation in general, and might reduce fibromyalgia pain, as well as uterine cramping associated with menstruation.

What You Should Know

Your doctor can test your blood to see whether you have adequate levels of vitamin D. In some cases, supplementation will not be beneficial unless you have an actual deficiency. With regard to dosing, recommendations vary depending on the health condition studied. In general, the recommended daily intake is 400 IU. In studies with participants who had fibromyalgia, doses typically ranged from 1200 IU to 2400 IU daily, although in at least one trial the dose was considerably higher. Dosing for fibromyalgia patients was determined based on the blood levels of vitamin D at the start of the trial. In studies of frail elderly patients, the dose has typically ranged from 800 to 1000 IU. Although some studies have used much larger doses for a variety of health conditions, too much vitamin D has been associated with increased risk of fractures, cardiovascular disease, cancer, and death. Therefore, your current blood test results and your doctor's guidance should determine how much D, if any, you decide to take.

Glucosamine, Chondroitin, and MSM

Glucosamine, chondroitin, and MSM (methylsulfonylmethane) are naturally occurring substances found in the body and are building blocks of cartilage. Glucosamine and chondroitin are also among the most frequently purchased dietary supplements in the United States, are often found in the same product, and sometimes are combined with MSM. With regard to glucosamine and chondroitin, the NCCIH has stated that the research on these substances has been conflicting and positive results have not warranted recommending the use of either supplement for reducing osteoarthritis pain or rebuilding cartilage.

This conclusion is in contrast to the findings from non-U.S. studies showing some reduction in joint narrowing in those who took a combination of glucosamine sulfate and chondroitin for knee osteoarthritis. Some findings suggest the *form* of glucosamine may determine whether it's helpful (the sulfate form being better than the hydrochloride form). For example, a 2015 study by Australian researchers at the University of Sidney found that taking glucosamine sulfate (1500 mg) plus chondroitin sulfate (800 mg) once daily for two years reduced the degree of knee-joint narrowing at the two-year follow-up. There was no significant benefit for joint narrowing taking either supplement alone, and there was no effect on pain for either the individual or combined supplements.

With regard to hand osteoarthritis, the data from a 2011 study by Swiss researchers suggests that taking 800 mg of chondroitan sulfate once daily is associated with reduced pain and improved function. At this time, there is not enough research on MSM to recommend it for joint pain or narrowing.

What You Should Know

Glucosamine and chondroitin are generally considered safe, however, they can interact with blood-thinning drugs, affect blood sugar, and at high doses over long periods of time may harm the kidneys. There is too little research on MSM to establish its safety. Side effects of MSM include skin rashes, digestive upset, and potential allergic reactions.

FACT

Although both D_2 and D_3 supplements are readily available and inexpensive, the current thinking is that D_3 is more effective at raising blood levels of 25-hydroxyvitamin D and may have greater therapeutic value.

Probiotics

Probiotics are bacteria that naturally occur in your digestive tract. Probiotic supplements contain mixes of probiotic bacteria and sometimes yeasts. They have gotten a significant amount of attention as of late, and for good reasons. They are included here because of their role in maintaining good overall health, and because the right balance of gut bacteria has been shown to be essential to balanced mood, good immune functioning, maintaining a healthy weight, and of course, optimal digestive functioning. Often, the balance of "good" bacteria becomes upset by the use of antibiotics, stress, and poor diet.

When the good bacteria are depleted, "bad" bacteria can overgrow and lead to chronic digestive problems (or worsen pre-existing ones), vaginal or other yeast infections, eczema, weight gain, anxiety, and depression.

QUESTION

Should probiotics be refrigerated?
Most probiotics require refrigeration and should be kept dry and away from heat. This is because heat can kill the organisms and moisture can activate them prematurely, making them ineffective. Probiotics that are freeze-dried don't have to be refrigerated but do need to be kept away from heat.

There are many, many strains of bacteria that can be included in probiotic supplements, and it can be confusing to determine which probiotic may be best for you. A number of studies have found some benefit of taking probiotics for symptoms of IBS such as gas, bloating, straining, diarrhea, and pain. The benefits varied depending on the types of bacteria included in the supplement.

The types that have been linked to reduction in gastrointestinal pain specifically in different studies are *Bifidobacterium infantis*, *Saccharomyces cerevisiae*, *L.* (for lactobacillus) *rhamnosus*, *L. plantarum*, *L. acidophilus*, *Enterococcum faeculis*, *L. reuteri*, and *L. casei*. Note that the combinations of bacteria and amounts varied across studies. It may take several weeks of taking a probiotic to notice a difference in GI pain, and this effect may not last after stopping the supplement. Doses have tended to range from 100 million to about 4 billion cells, and anything in this range should be safe.

With regard to mood benefits, 3 billion cells of *Bifidobacterium longum* and *L. helveticus* have been shown to reduce anxiety and depression.

What You Should Know

Probiotics are generally considered safe when purchased from a reputable manufacturer and used at the recommended doses on the labels. Because the types and doses available range greatly, speak with your doctor about the strains that are most likely to benefit you, given your medical issues and particular symptoms, or visit an independent laboratory such as Consumerlab.com for reviews and recommendations.

Magnesium

Magnesium is an essential mineral that is typically sold either alone or paired with calcium, or calcium and zinc. Magnesium can also be found in several compound supplements aimed at migraine relief. Certain illnesses such as digestive disorders, medications such as acid-blocking drugs and diuretics, and lifestyle behaviors such as excessive alcohol intake can lead to a magnesium deficiency. Low magnesium can lead to painful muscle spasms, insomnia, seizures, and irregular heartbeat, among other problems.

Magnesium supplementation has been used to manage insomnia, decrease migraines, alleviate constipation, and decrease pain associated with menstruation.

What You Should Know

Magnesium citrate has been shown to reduce the frequency and severity of migraines in doses of 600 mg once daily. Magnesium is thought to relax the nervous system and help with sleep, thus it is recommended to take it in the evening. Taking too much magnesium can cause stomach upset and diarrhea. Taking it with a meal reduces the likelihood of diarrhea. To help with sleep or menstrual cramps, begin with 250 mg of magnesium and increase up to 600 mg if no benefit is seen at lower doses.

Note that excessive intake of magnesium can lead to serious side effects, including death. If you have kidney disease, do not take magnesium without consulting your physician first. Because magnesium (and calcium) can interfere with the absorption of other vitamin/mineral supplements, take them at different times.

Capsaicin

Capsaicin is the ingredient in hot peppers (such as cayenne, jalapeño, and habanero) that makes them spicy. Capsaicin is also available in powder form, oral supplements, and topical preparations. Capsaicin works in a very interesting way in that although it causes a burning, painful sensation when eaten or applied to the skin, this sensation decreases over time.

A capsaicin cream is FDA approved for treating postherpetic neuralgia, a painful condition that can occur after having shingles. There is also evidence that topical capsaicin can help with diabetic peripheral neuropathy, and may help ease pain associated with fibromyalgia, minor indigestion, back pain, itching and discomfort associated with psoriasis, and protect the stomach from anti-inflammatory medications. If you have a gastrointestinal disorder, such as Crohn's disease or IBS, however, you may find that spicy food aggravates your symptoms. When in doubt, consult with your doctor.

FACT

Despite causing an initial burning sensation, capsaicin triggers the release of substance P, which is a chemical in your tissues responsible for causing the sensation of pain. Over time, applying capsaicin will further deplete substance P from an area and thus reduce the potential for pain. This is also why some people get used to eating extremely spicy food!

What You Should Know

In addition to helping manage pain, capsaicin is an antioxidant and may help prevent bacterial infections. Capsaicin is generally considered safe; however, use care when handling the powder form or preparing hot peppers; wear gloves, and don't allow either the powder or insides of peppers to come into contact with broken skin (same goes for the topical cream). Avoid touching your eyes or other mucus membranes after handling the cream or powder, or preparing peppers.

Omega-3 Fatty Acids

Omega-3s are found in higher concentrations in fatty fish such as mackerel, tuna, sea bass, and sardines, as well as in walnuts and flaxseeds. Omega-3s, because they reduce inflammation, are important for pain management and good overall health. There is also scientific support for omega-3's usefulness in reducing symptoms of depression and possibly for reducing situational anxiety. For most people, obtaining about 500 mg per day, whether from foods or supplements, can be beneficial, although you may experience a benefit with less. You'll notice on the labels of supplements that they will contain EPA (eicosapentaenoic acid), DHA (docosahexaenoic acid), or both. Although the research has shown antidepressant benefits for both types of oils, the combination of EPA and DHA, with EPA making up the greater percentage, seems to be better. The dosage in studies of depression has ranged widely, but it appears that taking somewhere between 1,000 and 2500 mg daily has been linked to a better effect.

A Swedish study of over thirty-two thousand women found that eating the equivalent of one meal per week of fatty fish such as salmon or four meals per week of leaner fish was associated with a 29 percent reduced risk of developing rheumatoid arthritis. Higher intakes of omega-3s from fish were linked to an over 50 percent reduction in RA risk. These effects were seen over the long term, after eating fish regularly for about seven and a half years.

What You Should Know

Because of environmental pollution, fish and fish oils can contain high levels of mercury. In addition, fish oil supplements can "repeat" on some people, leading to fishy-tasting burps. Supplements that are molecularly distilled have been purified to remove any potential contaminants, including mercury, and have no fishy taste. Note that fish oils from supplements decrease blood clotting, which can be a problem for those either taking blood thinners or having surgery. Excessively high doses may suppress immune function and lower blood pressure slightly. In addition, fish oil from supplements and fish may interfere with chemotherapy. If you are undergoing cancer treatment, discuss whether you should discontinue eating fish or consuming fish oils in the days right before and after chemotherapy.

Spices

Ginger is a plant native to southeastern Asia and a centuries-old remedy used for treating nausea and indigestion. More recently it has been examined for its potential benefit in reducing the pain of osteoarthritis and migraines. The evidence for ginger's effectiveness on both pain and nausea has been somewhat mixed, although this may be due to differences in the quality of the ginger used in different studies.

Ginger is generally recognized as safe, and many people report experiencing some benefit from using it. With regard to migraines, in a 2013 study of 100 migraine patients, a dose of 250 mg of dried ginger was found to be equally as helpful as the drug sumatriptan at reducing migraine severity. Specifically, more than half of those taking either the drug or ginger saw a 90 percent or greater reduction in migraine severity two hours after taking these treatments. Side effects were considerably less in the ginger group.

Ginger is also considered a warming, soothing herb and enhances the flavors of many foods. Raw ginger can be added to stir-fries and other cooked foods, and you can make a tea from a small piece of raw ginger root by peeling and submerging it in boiling water for a few minutes. Ginger is also sold as an encapsulated powder and in prepackaged herbal teas. If you are taking ginger for nausea or pain, start with 1 gram twice daily. You can increase up to 4 grams twice daily if no benefit is seen at a lower dose.

Ginger may decrease blood clotting, so speak with your doctor before taking it if you have a clotting disorder or are taking blood thinners. Ginger side effects, when they occur, are typically gas, bloating, heartburn, and nausea. These effects are usually associated with powdered rather than fresh ginger.

Turmeric

Turmeric is a shrub related to ginger and is grown in India, other parts of Asia, and Africa. It produces an orange-colored spice that is also found in condiments like curry powder. There is some evidence that the active ingredient, curcumin, can help alleviate symptoms of indigestion, may help those who have ulcerative colitis remain in remission for longer, may reduce joint swelling and stiffness in those who have rheumatoid arthritis, and may also help reduce pain and improve function in those with osteoarthritis.

There is also some evidence that curcumin may improve depression symptoms when added to an antidepressant regimen and may improve cognitive functioning and short-term, but not long-term, memory in the elderly.

Preliminary findings from animal studies suggest that turmeric may reduce inflammation and also may have anticancer and antioxidant properties. Current research is under way to see if turmeric may help prevent liver cancer and other illnesses.

The doses of the spice turmeric and the active ingredient curcumin used in research have been higher than what you would likely obtain via diet alone. Some studies have looked at the spice powder, some at curcumin alone, and some have combined curcumin with other ingredients. Therefore, it is difficult to recommend specific doses; however, therapeutic doses in studies have ranged between 500 and 2,000 mg. Daily intakes higher than 500 mg have tended to be divided into 500 mg doses.

According to the NCCIH, turmeric is considered safe for most adults, but high doses can cause indigestion, nausea, or diarrhea, and in animal studies have caused liver problems. No liver problems have been reported in humans. Turmeric may worsen gallbladder symptoms or disease.

Vitamin B_{12} and Folate

B vitamins, such as B_{12} and folate, are essential for healthy nervous system functioning and stable mood. Although deficiencies are less likely with a well-balanced diet, some medical conditions, lifestyle behaviors, and medications can reduce the body's ability to adequately use either vitamin even if you are consuming enough. For example, those with digestive or eating disorders, or who consume excessive alcohol can become B vitamin deficient. Certain types of chemotherapy, anticonvulsant medications, diabetes drugs, and acid-reducing medications can inhibit absorption of B_{12} or folate. In addition, a type of genetic mutation (MTHFR) is linked to significantly reduced ability to use B_{12} and folate, and is also linked to greater risk of having migraines, depression, and other health issues.

Signs of severe B vitamin deficiency include fatigue, muscle weakness, diarrhea, difficulty concentrating, forgetfulness, sleeplessness, irritability, depression, and anxiety. In very severe cases, deficiency can result in seizures, dementia, or paresthesia (burning, prickling, tingling, numbness, or a crawling sensation in the extremities or elsewhere in the body).

Low levels of B_{12} and folate are also associated with having higher levels of homocysteine, an amino acid found in the blood; when homocysteine levels are too high, the risks of cardiovascular disease and cognitive problems increase.

L-methylfolate, the most bioavailable type of folate supplement, has been shown to improve the response to antidepressant medications and in some cases has alleviated depression sufficiently to discontinue other treatments. More recent research has found that L-methylfolate supplementation can enhance the repair of nerve tissues and, pending further study, may be of significant benefit for those suffering from brain and spinal cord injuries and other damage to neurons.

What You Should Know

B_{12} and folate deficiencies can be difficult to tell apart, and high doses of folate supplementation can mask a B_{12} deficiency. Therefore, it is recommended to also take B_{12} when taking folate supplements. In addition, you can have adequate blood levels of either or both vitamins, but if you have one of the issues linked to poor absorption, test results may be misleading. Using the more bioavailable forms of these vitamins, L-methylfolate (folate) and methylcobalamin (B_{12}), typically yields better results than the forms commonly added to vitamins and fortified foods (folic acid and cyanocobalamin).

B vitamins are water soluble, meaning that you will likely excrete in your urine anything beyond what your body needs. In general, 400 mcg of L-methylfolate and 400 mcg daily of methylcobalamin should be sufficient to help maintain good general health. If you have been diagnosed with diabetic peripheral neuropathy, your doctor may prescribe a supplement combining considerably higher amounts of these vitamins. If you are severely B_{12} deficient, or have a medical condition that interferes with your body's ability to use the oral form, you may require B_{12} injections or higher oral doses of folate and B_{12}.

Folic acid supplementation has become somewhat controversial in recent years. Some studies have suggested that this vitamin may protect against colorectal cancer, but recently there has been some concern that excessive folic acid supplementation may slightly increase the growth of some other cancers. Yet, a large meta-analysis of studies including over 49,000 patients found no effect at all of folic acid supplementation on cancer risk. The take-away message is that if you have symptoms of B vitamin deficiency or are at high risk for one, speak with your doctor about whether and how much to supplement.

Although B vitamins are generally safe, they can interact with other medications. Finally, you should not discontinue using prescribed antidepressants or other psychiatric medications without consulting your physician, as doing so can result in sudden and significant worsening of symptoms.

FACT

MTHFR is the acronym for both a gene and the essential enzyme it is involved in producing. MTHFR mutations can reduce the enzyme's ability to use B vitamins for a number of bodily processes. This can lead to elevated homocysteine levels, increased risk of certain illnesses, and impaired cognitive and emotional functioning. For more information on MTHFR, visit the National Institutes of Health: http://ghr.nlm.nih.gov/gene/MTHFR.

Eric and the "Perfect Storm"

Eric was a single father in his 30s who had received a diagnosis of Crohn's disease in his 20s and continued to struggle ten years later. He continued to have flare-ups with the bouts of diarrhea, abdominal pain, low energy, and body aches common to those with this illness. Eric took his medications as prescribed, including an acid-blocking medication to alleviate symptoms of gastroesophageal reflux. He also took a daily multivitamin. Despite his best efforts to eat well, Eric noticed that his appetite tended to vary, and when he was especially busy with his children or work projects, his eating became more irregular and he lost a considerable amount of weight, as he sometime did when experiencing a flare-up.

Over time, Eric noticed that he felt increasingly lethargic and down, depressed despite the lack of an obvious emotional trigger, and had greater difficulty remaining focused at work. Antidepressant medications seemed to have limited effect these issues.

When Eric began to notice odd and painful pins and needles sensations in his hands and arms, he became especially worried. His gastroenterologist was unable to find a reason for his symptoms and referred him first to a neurologist, who could find nothing to explain Eric's symptoms, leaving Eric feeling more frustrated and worried than ever.

Eric eventually consulted with an integrative pain specialist. After examining Eric and running blood tests, the doctor told Eric, "I think I may know what's causing or at least contributing to your symptoms." He diagnosed Eric with an MTHFR mutation and also said he thought the acid blocker was causing a problem with B vitamin absorption. "Your blood levels of folate and B_{12} are actually normal, probably due to your taking a multivitamin, but I don't think your body is able to use these sufficiently, given the combination of Crohn's, the acid blocker, and the MTHFR." The doctor prescribed a high-dose supplement containing L-methylfolate, methylcobalamin, and B_6. Within about a month, Eric noticed the pins and needles had ceased and that his mood, appetite, energy levels, and thinking were much improved.

CHAPTER 9

Biofeedback and Binaural Beat Technology

Everyone has bodily functions that are *voluntary*, such as deciding to walk and then taking a step forward. *Involuntary* functions include heart rate, blood pressure, digestion, and whether your predominant brain wave patterns reflect anxiety, relaxation, or another state. Yet, since the 1960s, biofeedback has been used to train people to gain conscious control over many involuntary functions to help them feel increased calm and less pain. Binaural beat technology, like EEG biofeedback, can also facilitate changes in your brain to increase relaxation, improve sleep, and enhance well-being.

What Is Biofeedback?

Biofeedback refers to the process of a computer monitoring and providing information about your body's responses to internal stimuli and external stimuli. The term "internal stimuli" refers to your thoughts and emotions, memories, and so forth. These things are absolutely able to influence your heart rate, blood pressure, how much you perspire, and how tense your muscles are. They also impact whether your brain responds by paying attention, becoming distracted, or reflecting increased anxiety.

The term "external stimuli" simply refers to anything outside you that can generate a particular response in your body or mind. For example, if you bump into a piece of furniture while walking and you feel pain, the injury is a type of *external* stimulus that causes an *internal* response—such as the sensation of pain or the thought, "Why wasn't I watching where I was going?" Other types of external stimuli that are relevant to pain and distress could include listening to music that is soothing (and then feeling more relaxed as a result) or placing a hot water bottle over your belly to soothe abdominal cramps.

How Biofeedback Works

The feedback part of biofeedback encourages you to provide a response that will result in a "reward" of some sort. The computer's feedback motivates you to change the way your body or mind responds to something. This process is referred to as operant conditioning. You may have heard this term in the context of behavior therapy. Operant conditioning refers to learning occurring as a result of receiving some sort of reward (or punishment) from the environment. The environment can mean a person, such as when your boss, a friend, or teacher praises you for a job well done. The environment can also refer to something like an object, such as a slot machine at a casino that rewards you for putting money in again and again by (eventually) paying out a jackpot.

As an example, if your boss (the environment) gave you a raise for each instance that you were on time for work, your brain would make the connection between a specific response (being on time) and a reward (an increase in your pay). Because people are hard-wired to seek pleasurable outcomes, receiving raises for timely arrival to work would probably increase the likelihood of your being on time. (Although punishment is also used in operant conditioning as a way of discouraging an undesirable behavior, it is thankfully not used in biofeedback!)

FACT

Biofeedback is used to treat a number of health-related issues, including tension headaches, migraines, lower back pain, temporomandibular joint disorders, hypertension, Raynaud's disease, incontinence, and a number of other functional disorders. It has also been used to treat addictions, improve sleep, and decrease reactivity to stress.

In the case of biofeedback, the environment refers to signals from a computer program telling you that you have reached a goal. These signals could come in the form of music playing, a tone sounding, or animation changing every time you successfully decrease tension in a muscle group, slow your heart rate, decrease perspiration, slow your respiration rate, or decrease your blood pressure—all signs of relaxation. Biofeedback offers many ways to train the body and mind, and the feedback from the sensors to the computer, and thus to your brain, is virtually instantaneous.

The Biofeedback Session

Biofeedback is offered in a variety of settings, including hospitals, freestanding biofeedback clinics, and in the private practice offices of psychologists, physicians, independent biofeedback technicians, and other healthcare providers. Biofeedback is also offered in some specialized pain centers, including headache centers, spine medicine services, and departments of rehabilitation medicine. A biofeedback session typically ranges from thirty minutes to one hour, may take place within the context of psychotherapy (if provided by a psychologist), and may or may not be covered by your insurance.

Biofeedback has been shown to decrease symptoms of anxiety and depression and reduce pain severity for a number of conditions. Although the electronic feedback is delivered via computer, the therapist or technician will likely provide guidance, support, and instruction as needed.

FACT

Although biofeedback on its own is an effective treatment for many symptoms, it is very often used in conjunction with other mind-body techniques such as mindfulness, imagery, self-hypnosis, or diaphragmatic breathing. The ultimate goal is to elicit the same response outside of sessions.

There are many types of biofeedback sensors and modalities. The following are descriptions of the most commonly used types of biofeedback. Very often a biofeedback session will combine more than one type:

- **EMG**, or electromyography, involves sensing the degree of tension in a specific muscle group and reporting changes in this tension. EMG is especially helpful for a number of chronic pain conditions. Painless sensors are attached to the skin in various locations, and the computer registers when tension is over or under a predetermined threshold. EMG is useful for treating both migraine and tension-type headaches, TMJ, muscle spasms, and back and neck pain. EMG can also be used to strengthen muscles, as in the case of urinary incontinence.
- **Thermal**, or temperature, biofeedback involves attaching a tiny sensor, usually to a fingertip, to measure changes in temperature. Just as your muscles tense when you are under stress, your blood vessels constrict in response to emotional tension, decreasing peripheral blood flow and resulting in a drop in temperature in your extremities (hands and feet). Conversely, increasing relaxation will cause a rapid rise in temperature in these areas. Thermal biofeedback is useful for general relaxation training as well as for those who have Raynaud's disease, or who experience peripheral skin temperature changes due to CRPS, have hypertension, or experience migraine headaches.
- **Galvanic skin response** biofeedback, or GSR, involves using sensors that measure the activity of your sweat glands and the amount of perspiration on your skin. Increased perspiration is associated with greater anxiety, and vice versa. GSR can detect extremely small changes in perspiration—much smaller changes than you might notice on your own. GSR has been used to reduce seizure frequency in patients with epilepsy, treat tension-type headache, and in general is effective for decreasing stress and increasing relaxation.

- **Blood Volume Pulse** (BVP) biofeedback has been less well studied than the types already listed, but more evidence is emerging with regard to its potential therapeutic value. The BVP sensor is wrapped around the tip of a finger and monitors the blood flow in your arteries, providing feedback about heart rate variability (HRV) and other related measures. The basic premise of HRV is that the healthy heart has sufficient HRV to adapt to the demands placed upon it. For example, your heart rate should be quite a bit slower when you are sitting and reading a book than when you are sprinting to catch a bus, and vice versa. HRV is commonly paired with a sensor that measures respiration rate. A respiration sensor is useful for training you to breathe slowly and deeply, facilitating relaxation. As with the other sensors, respiration biofeedback can be used on its own or with other types of biofeedback. HRV has been found to be effective for decreasing functional abdominal pain, enhancing migraine management, and improving pain and depression related to fibromyalgia. BVP is more difficult to interpret than other types of biofeedback, however, and this may be why it is less commonly used.

- **EEG** biofeedback, otherwise known as neurofeedback, involves the placement of sensors at one or more locations on your scalp for the purposes of assessing and entraining brain wave activity. Neurofeedback makes the spectrum of brain waves "visible" via a computer screen. You always have a variety of different types of brain wave activity, but usually one or two frequencies will predominate, indicating something about your brain's functioning at any given time. Briefly, medium-fast brain wave activity (beta) is associated with being awake and alert and paying attention. Somewhat slower activity (alpha) is associated with being awake but relaxed, and perhaps a bit daydreamy, or in a light state of meditation. Even slower still are theta brain waves, which are associated with deeper meditation and light sleep. Very deep, dreamless sleep is associated with the slowest type of brain waves, referred to as delta. High-beta brain waves are faster than typical beta brain waves and are associated with anxiety and pain.

Neurofeedback enables you to know what your predominant brain wave activity is in the present moment and train your brain to achieve a desired state. Much like with heart rate variability, there is no "wrong" brainwave state, but rather, ideally you want your brain to be in the predominant brain wave state that corresponds to the type of task at hand.

With regard to pain, this may mean training to achieve what is referred to as sensorimotor or SMR brain wave activity, which is slower than beta but faster than alpha. SMR has been linked to improved attention and decreased impulsivity in those who have attention deficit disorder, as well as decreased insomnia and enhanced calm. Alpha and theta training are also used to reduce pain and increase calm.

FACT

Neurofeedback and biofeedback have been shown to help with migraine management, attention, and sleep, among other issues. Although biofeedback and neurofeedback are typically used as therapeutic training tools, they can also shed light on what external and internal events tend to trigger pain and mood symptoms.

Harry—Biofeedback and the "Aha" Moment

Harry was a very shy but successful college student who suffered from temporomandibular joint pain (TMJ). He experienced limited relief from either the medical or other relaxation therapies he had tried, and sought out treatment with biofeedback. Harry was aware of many triggers of his pain, including anxiety prior to exams, when he was sleep deprived, and when he slept on one side for too long. After keeping a pain diary, however, Harry also became aware that his pain worsened significantly in December, right before the Christmas break, and typically lessened as he returned to school in January.

"I just don't get why my pain should increase when I've finished my finals. I'll get to visit my family and friends from home, have some terrific home-cooked meals for a few weeks, and won't have any homework to do." Harry reportedly got along well with his family—a large group of close-knit people who were very supportive of him. It didn't make sense to him that his pain should spike.

After a few sessions, Harry learned to relax his face and jaw via EMG bio-feedback. At the fifth session, when Harry was hooked up to a temperature sensor, however, it became clear that going home was more stressful for him than he realized. In particular, Harry's temperature dropped dramatically when he described how chatty and outgoing everyone else in his family was compared to him, and how self-conscious he felt about having to be "funny" or "engaging" on demand in order to fit in. He also noticed that he had a much greater need for privacy and quiet than his siblings did, and disliked having to share a room with two of his five brothers when he went home.

"It's weird, but I never thought about being stressed and having more pain from things that are also good in some way—like spending time with my family. But I really do need some space when I'm home—they are just way louder than I can deal with twenty-four hours, seven days a week, and it just gets to be way, way too much."

This information was invaluable in helping Harry pinpoint important triggers of pain, anxiety, and frustration, and helped him further realize the importance of practicing stress management techniques ahead of time to help him cope once in a busy, loud household. Harry also was able to reframe his shyness as an individual difference, and thus felt less pressured to try to be like everyone else in his family to be "okay." Finally, Harry was able to negotiate sleeping in a smaller bedroom with only one brother— the next quietest one in the bunch—who wound up spending several nights at a friend's house during Harry's stay. This situation provided Harry with some much-needed quiet so he could better tolerate the festivities the rest of the time. Harry later noted that biofeedback had helped him both elicit the relaxation response more consciously and also to make changes that helped him feel less stressed and therefore have reduced pain for the first visit home in a while.

FACT

The "fight or flight" response is the opposite of the relaxation response and leads to increased heart rate, breathing, and blood pressure. Fight or flight is useful if you must flee from a dangerous situation or fight your way out of it, but otherwise it's associated with increased risk of health problems, stress, and more severe pain.

The Importance of At-Home Practice

As with many of the other therapies discussed in this book, biofeedback is most effective when also practiced at home, in between sessions, in addition to in the provider's office. At-home practice can take any of several forms.

Relaxation Training

Whatever relaxation technique is paired with biofeedback during your sessions can be practiced on its own in a variety of other settings—at home, during a brief break while at work or school, and even while falling asleep. You will learn more about specific techniques in other chapters, but diaphragmatic breathing, mindfulness, progressive muscle relaxation, guided imagery, and self-hypnosis can be practiced with minimal or no equipment, and can train the brain and body to increase feelings of peace and comfort and decrease stress. The more you practice, the more easily and rapidly you will elicit and recognize the relaxation response.

At-Home Biofeedback Devices

There are a number of at-home biofeedback devices available, ranging from using an "old-school" thermometer as a temperature sensor, to portable temperature, blood pressure, respiration rate, and GSR biofeedback devices. There are also computer software programs that train the brain and body similarly to what is offered in-office.

The prices of at-home equipment can range from a few dollars for a thermometer to between $20 and $150 for a small stand-alone device, a few hundred dollars for biofeedback software, and closer to a thousand dollars for the newest at-home EEG headsets with software. Granted, even the most expensive of these is considerably less than the thousands of dollars one would pay for professional equipment and training. Cost aside, by far the most important factor with regard to selection of an at-home biofeedback device is whether or not you are likely to use regularly whatever you purchase. If you will use a one-dollar disposable thermometer regularly, that will be more valuable to you than the thousand-dollar EEG headset that remains in its box.

Biofeedback Apps

There are a variety of apps that can enable you to use your smartphone as a biofeedback device or to otherwise practice relaxation techniques. For the most part, the apps range from free to low cost.

- MyCalmBeat is a free app available for iOS, Android, Blackberry, and online. It trains you to breathe slowly and deeply, facilitating relaxation and indirectly decreasing heart rate and blood pressure. For more information, visit *www.mybrainsolutions.com/mycalmbeat*.
- Ambience is an app for iOS and Android that at this writing is $2.99. The app aims to help you create a desired ambient sound—whether to relax or focus. It also allows you to record your own sounds, play sounds in the background, and mix in your own music. Choose from a number of free sounds or purchase premium ones. Visit *http://ambianceapp.com*.
- Sleep Pillow is a free app for iOS that provides over eighty soothing nature sounds to help with sleep and relaxation. It also features an alarm clock and sleep timer for napping. Visit *https://itunes.apple.com/us/app/sleep-pillow-sounds-white/id410606661?mt=8*.
- Instant Heart Rate—Heart Rate Monitor by Azumio is an app for IOS, Android, and the Windows phone that measures—you guessed it—heart rate, using your phone's camera. It also tracks trends over time. At this writing it costs $1.99 and utilizes your smartphone's camera to obtain heart rate data. Visit *www.azumio.com/s/instantheartrate/index.html*.
- Mindfield eSense Temperature is a free app for IOS and Android; however, it requires the purchase of a device that costs $99. The same company also makes free apps that enable your phone to be used for GSR and HRV biofeedback. These, too, require the purchase of relevant devices, for $99 and $129, respectively. Visit *http://bio-medical.com* for more information.

Finding a Biofeedback Provider

Biofeedback can be provided by a licensed psychologist who is specifically trained to administer biofeedback. Other types of health professionals can be certified to use biofeedback in clinical practice. One resource for locating certified biofeedback providers is The Association for Applied Psychophysiology and Biofeedback (*www.aapb.org*). Another is the Biofeedback Certification International Alliance (*www.bcia.org*). The American Psychological Association (*www.APA.org*) and state psychological associations maintain referral databases that can be searched for psychologists who offer biofeedback and stress management and who work with chronic pain issues.

Binaural Beat Technology

Binaural beat technology (BBT) does not provide the "feedback" that biofeedback does. Yet it is an inexpensive and easy-to-use approach that may help increase well-being. BBT was discovered in the early 1800s and first described in popular literature in the early 1970s. In recent years, binaural beat audio programs have been touted as tools for reducing stress, improving sleep, enhancing concentration, decreasing headache pain, and even fostering altered states of consciousness. Although the prevalence and popularity of such products has waxed and waned, several studies have examined the potential usefulness of BBT for a variety of issues.

What Is BBT?

The term "binaural beat" refers to the brain's tendency to hear the difference between two similar tones that are played in opposite ears as one new tone. Your ears hear tones in terms of hertz (Hz), or cycles (the number of times a wave repeats itself) per second. So if you were to hear a 100 Hz tone in your right ear and a 102 Hz tone in your left ear, your brain would register hearing a tone of 2 Hz, because 102 minus 100 is two. Beats played at frequencies that are characteristic of brain wave frequencies are both audible and thought to change the predominant brain wave state. For example, a resulting tone of 2 Hz would shift your predominant brain wave pattern to delta (that of deep sleep).

FACT

Typically, the BBT audio programs you will find today, packaged as MP3 or on CDs, will feature another sound, such as music or ocean waves, to camouflage the BBT tones. Theoretically, your brain will hear the difference in hertz even if you do not consciously register that you are hearing the BBT.

Alpha, Beta, Theta . . . Oh My!

Brain wave frequencies are each categorized according to a particular range of hertz and the cognitive states associated with these ranges. For example:

- Deep, dreamless sleep is referred to as "delta," which ranges from 1–4 Hz
- "Theta," which ranges from 4–8 Hz, is the predominant brain wave of light to medium sleep, and deeper states of meditation
- "Alpha" (8–12 Hz) is a state of relaxed awareness or daydreaming, or relaxed focus
- The "beta" range includes the subcategories of low beta, or what is known as sensorimotor rhythm (SMR; 12–15 Hz), which is experienced as comfortable but alert awareness; mid beta, which falls within 15–18 Hz and characterizes alert mental activity and focused concentration; and high beta, which ranges from >18 Hz to about 39 Hz, and can be indicative of anxiety or "hyper-arousal" such as after ingesting caffeine or another stimulant
- Gamma brainwaves (40 Hz and above) are the least well studied of the brain wave frequencies; however, they are thought to be associated with higher mental activity, such as relaxed but intense focus and feelings of transcendence, love, and peace.

There is no "best" predominant brain wave state to be in. At different times you will understandably want to be able to shift into one that is appropriate to the task at hand, whether sleeping, working on a project, meditating, or relaxing. Thus, if you are taking an exam, you will want the predominant brain wave state to be mid beta to facilitate enhanced concentration without feeling jittery. For deep sleep, a BBT program that gradually induces a predominance of theta and then delta waves will be most useful. And to enhance relaxation and creativity without making you sleepy, an alpha or gamma state is the way to go.

It has been suggested that a number of conditions, including chronic stress, chronic and postoperative pain, migraines and other headaches, problems with attention/concentration or learning, and insomnia, reflect an imbalance or irregularity in brain wave states. The deliberate use of BBT to change the predominant brain wave state is referred to as brain wave entrainment (BWE).

FACT

The Monroe Institute produces "Hemi-Sync" programs that feature BBT and other sounds. Hemi-Sync may improve general well-being, provide some degree of pain relief, and reduce feelings of anxiety. In general, users report feeling relaxed and peaceful after listening. More research is needed to better understand how and with what issues Hemi-Sync may be helpful.

What's the Evidence for BBT?

A 2008 review of the BWE literature found that delta stimulation was associated with improvement in migraines and other headaches and reduction in short-term stress. A single session of alpha stimulation was associated with stress reduction in some settings, and alpha stimulation was also linked to pain relief. Mid-beta improved attention, reduced short-term stress, alleviated headaches, reduced behavioral problems, and improved performance on measures of overall intelligence.

BBT for Reducing Anxiety and Pain

A 2005 study found that listening to an audio program featuring BBT plus music could reduce anxiety in patients undergoing surgery with general anesthesia. Listening for thirty minutes preoperatively was more effective than listening to music alone or receiving no intervention at all. In this study, the BBT audio featured a progressively slowing beat that ended with ten minutes of delta wave-inducing tones.

None of the participants in this study reported any adverse effects from BBT. This study showed that an inexpensive, one-time intervention of short duration was beneficial, despite the stress characteristic of undergoing surgery.

Another study of BBT involved patients who were about to have surgery under general anesthesia. Twenty patients were assigned to each of three conditions: a Hemi-Sync BBT program, listening to the music of their choosing, or listening to a blank audiocassette, for thirty minutes prior to surgery. None of the participants was offered any sedative premedication. The researchers found that using the Hemi-Sync programs resulted in significantly less use of fentanyl (a potent, synthetic opioid pain medication) during surgery, lower self-reported pain scores several hours after the surgery, and being discharged from the hospital sooner. Unfortunately, the specific frequency of BBT was not described in this article.

FACT

APPCRAWLR is a site that provides comparison charts of iPhone and Android apps, including ones for a binaural beats and ambient sound. It lists the prices, types of sounds offered, goals targeted, and other features you may want to know about before trying a particular app. This chart also indicates the average customer rating and popularity of individual apps. Visit *http://appcrawlr.com*.

Binaural Beat Technology Apps

There are several free and inexpensive apps that feature either ambient sounds such as nature sounds or soothing music, BBT, or both. Some of these are geared more to enhancing relaxation or fostering deep sleep or meditative states, and others also include programs to enhance concentration and focus, as well as creativity. Isochronic tones are said to facilitate brain wave entrainment similarly to BBT, but without requiring the use of stereo headphones.

- Brainwave Studio is a low-fee iPhone app that uses isochronic tones. The app is easy to use and provides options for customizing programs in five broad categories: relaxation, reducing stress and anxiety, facilitating meditation, sleep, and "mind training." The last category features options to enhance concentration while you work, enhance sports performance, and encourage creativity, among other functions. For more information, visit *https://itunes.apple.com/us/app/brainwave-studio/id548229245?mt=12*.
- Isochronic & Binaural Beats is a popular and free Android app that uses both BBT and isochronic tones to facilitate relaxation and sleep. It also aims to improve concentration, deepen meditation, and

enhance learning, and is customizable. For more information, visit *https://play.google.com/store/apps/details?id=com.cpcapps.braindroid&hl+en*.

- Brain Wave - 32 Advanced Binaural Brainwave Entrainment Programs is a low-cost iPhone app that features a number of settings, including ones to alleviate a headache, reduce stress, cool anger, facilitate deep sleep, enhance meditation, and more. It is very customizable and allows you to choose from a range of ambient sounds, use with your own iTunes Music, and more. For more information, visit *https://itunes.apple.com/us/app/brain-wave-32-advanced-binaural/id307219387?mt=8*.

In summary, BBT has been available to the consumer for decades and is easily accessible and inexpensive. There is some data to suggest that BBT may be helpful for relieving anxiety and may help with pain, concentration, headaches, and other issues. Assuming BBT is effective, in general you should not drive or perform tasks requiring sharp focus when listening, and especially if the audio features delta, theta, or alpha tones, or is designed to help with sleep, deepen meditation, or otherwise induce a very relaxed state.

CHAPTER 10

Hypnosis and Guided Imagery

Guided imagery and hypnosis are two mind-body tools that have considerable evidence of benefit. Specifically, they can help with reducing acute and chronic pain, and decreasing distress, as well as with other issues. Imagery and hypnosis can be guided by a therapist or created and practiced on your own. There are also a number of imagery and hypnosis audio programs available for download. Both techniques draw upon your innate ability to "go within" and use your mind to turn the volume down on pain and feel better in general.

Two of the Most "Natural" Therapies

In childhood, long before you could even think about your own process of thinking (known as "metacognition"), you engaged in some form of imagery every single day. When you daydreamed about your mother baking your favorite cookies, your mind formed a flowing series of multisensory images. When you fantasized about receiving a particular toy for your birthday, your brain created a facsimile of what you imagined this experience would be like. And as the movie played in your mind about the treat or the toy, or perhaps getting the lead in the school play, you also experienced emotional, physical, and intellectual responses—for example, joy, hunger, longing, and perhaps impatience. Thus, the tendency to use the mind's imagery to change how you feel, or move your attention from one thing to another, is among the most natural and automatic things in the world.

FACT

Imagery and trance have been used since ancient times to achieve desired psychological and spiritual states. In the late 1950s, both the American Medical Association and the American Psychological Association recognized hypnotherapy as a valid medical treatment. The National Institutes of Health (NIH) has since recommended hypnotherapy as a treatment for chronic pain.

The Overlap Between Imagery and Hypnosis

Although they are not the same thing, imagery and hypnosis have some key features in common. First, both are "top-down" techniques that close the pain gate described in an earlier chapter. They accomplish this analgesic effect by decreasing distress, providing a pleasant distraction, inducing feelings of calm beyond what is achieved via normal types of relaxation (such as watching TV), and helping your brain reframe or change the meaning attributed to bodily sensations. All of these effects serve to send information down your spinal cord that changes the interpretation of signals coming from the peripheral nerves. The result is that hypnosis and imagery can partially or completely block pain and considerably decrease distress.

The terms imagery and hypnosis are often used interchangeably, and you will also likely hear the term "hypnotic imagery" when imagery is used for the purpose of inducing or shaping a particular trance. Because imagery shifts the bulk of your awareness inward, it tends to create a light hypnotic trance on its own; by definition, trance states shift the larger part of your focus to your inner world. This shift takes the forms of visual images, bodily sensations, sounds you "hear," remembered or imagined smells and tastes, a sense of temperature, movement, and so forth. And imagery can change the meaning you attribute to a feeling, thought, sensation, or situation, and thus can be particularly helpful if you tend to catastrophize or have significant anxiety about pain.

The Power of Everyday Imagery

Although therapeutic imagery is specifically designed to be healing, you actually experience your own imagery nearly constantly without even thinking about it. For example, if you were to hear a friend vividly describe the pizza he recently ate—the taste, mouth feel, and perhaps the crunchiness of the hot, crispy crust, the creamy melted cheese stretching in a long line before it breaks, the spicy aroma of oregano, the tangy tomato sauce—your own mouth would almost certainly water, particularly if you are hungry. In fact, advertisers make very good use of the fact that you will tend to create your own imagery to match what you hear someone saying or see someone else experiencing.

Your own mind will readily fill in the gaps that are left by that commercial for a "cool, refreshing" beverage, or the laundry detergent that smells "summertime fresh." An ad depicting a vacationing family frolicking in a crystal-clear pool or riding horseback on a powdery beach may stimulate your own longing to get away such that you wind up booking a similar trip soon afterward.

QUESTION

Will I embarrass myself if I undergo hypnosis?
Only if you choose to. All hypnosis is really self-hypnosis. So you will not quack like a duck or reveal your most deeply held secret unless some part of you truly wants to do this.

Imagery Is Hypnotic, but Hypnosis Is More than Imagery

Hypnosis is different from imagery in that it is characterized by being in a trance state—whether or not imagery is used to induce or shape the trance. Everyday hypnotic trances are brought on quite commonly by rhythmic activities such as dancing, driving, jogging, intense prayer, and even by having sex. A conversation with someone can trigger a type of trance state, as well, because your mind will form its own version of the story that the person across from you is describing. But again, trance, at its essence, is an intense state of inner focus, rather than focus on your external environment.

Your Brain and Hypnotic Imagery

As you now know, there are multiple brain areas involved in the experience of pain. Recent research conducted by Dr. Mark Jensen of the University of Washington, and other scientists, has found that not only does the brain respond to hypnotic suggestions, but that different areas of the brain respond depending on the type of suggestion. For example, hypnotic suggestions to decrease the unpleasantness of pain have been shown to decrease activity in the anterior cingulate cortex, or ACC. The ACC is located in the middle of the front part of the brain, and is involved in assigning a positive or negative emotional value to something you perceive.

As an example, suggestions to detach from pain sensations, noticing them as if you were simply a neutral observer, can decrease pain's unpleasantness. In addition, noticing areas of your body or mind that feel comfortable, or neutral, are ways to increase what feels good to you and also decrease pain's unpleasantness.

FACT

Hypnosis has been shown to cause measurable changes in inflammation, blood flow, and wound healing, and also to cause changes in brain activity that are visible on fMRI (functional magnetic resonance imaging). The effect of hypnosis is actually both very real and observable in both the brain and the body.

Hypnotic suggestions that emphasize reducing pain severity specifically decrease activity in the somatosensory areas of the brain. The somatosensory cortex is a strip that is located in roughly the middle of the outer layer of the brain, like a narrow headband. The somatosensory cortex tells you how severe the pain is, the quality of the sensation (such as sharp, dull throbbing, etc.), and where the pain is located.

There are several other areas involved in the creation of pain, but those just mentioned are the ones especially worth knowing about as you think about using hypnosis.

Clinical Hypnotherapy

The term clinical hypnotherapy refers to formal trances conducted within the context of psychotherapy. During a clinical hypnosis session, a trained hypnotherapist will guide you into a deeper state of relaxation and inner focus than you normally experience. Once you are sufficiently relaxed and comfortable, you will be more receptive to hypnotic suggestions that are consistent with your goals for treatment.

Hypnotists vs. Hypnotherapists

A "certified clinical hypnotherapist" is a person who is formally trained in the techniques and practice of hypnotherapy and also holds at least a master's level degree and is licensed to provide a clinical service separate from hypnosis. At this writing, psychologists, social workers, licensed professional counselors, physicians, dentists, and master's level nurses are eligible to become certified clinical hypnotherapists.

A "hypnotist" is simply someone who has learned to use hypnotic techniques to induce and shape trance, but is not necessarily a licensed healthcare provider. Someone may refer to himself as a hypnotist and have little to no formal training in hypnosis and no clinical training at all in a health-related field.

ALERT

The golden rule of hypnotherapy is to seek someone who would be qualified to treat your issue *even without the use of hypnosis*, such as a certified clinical hypnotherapist, rather than a hypnotist. One reason is because your pain, anxiety, depression, or other issue may or may not respond sufficiently to hypnosis alone.

In clinical hypnosis with a trained and licensed provider, the goals of hypnosis are explicitly discussed and agreed upon before any formal hypnosis takes place. The therapist is there to guide you, but *you* are ultimately in control. The hypnotherapist should also have in-depth, formal training in a healthcare discipline related to chronic pain, psychotherapy, etc., and adhere to his profession's code of ethics.

Emmy and the Ten-Year Tinnitus

Emmy had struggled with near constant tinnitus, or a bothersome and uncomfortable ringing in her ears, ever since a serious car accident she'd been in a decade earlier. Emmy had recovered from back and neck pain caused by the accident, but she continued to experience tinnitus despite consultation with several different doctors, a dentist, and treatment with acupuncture.

"I feel like I'm nearly at the end of my rope with this. Most people can't imagine living with a noise they can't turn off or block out. Day and night, when I'm trying to sleep, work, you name it, this whistling sound is driving me crazy!"

Emmy wanted to avoid taking medication as she was hoping to become pregnant within the year. She described herself as creative, open-minded, and curious by nature—all qualities that made her an excellent candidate for hypnosis. In her sessions, the hypnotic suggestions focused on increasing Emmy's ability to move her attention to both internal sensations, such as the feeling of warmth in her hands as they rested in her lap, as well as to external stimuli, such as the hum of the air conditioner. This practice would help her shift her attention away from the ringing at will. Emmy also received the specific suggestion for being able to turn down the volume on the ringing in her ears, just as she could turn down the volume on a radio or the TV in her normal daily life.

In addition to these suggestions, Emmy learned techniques for self-hypnosis that she could practice at home, such as focusing on her breathing, counting back from 100 to 1, and calling to mind an image of a quiet and peaceful lake surrounded by trees—a place that made her feel calm and wonderful each time she "went" there in her mind.

After a month, Emmy came into the session nearly bursting with excitement. "Guess what? I realized yesterday that there were times when *I didn't notice any ringing at all.* And in general, I've been a lot less bothered by the whistling sound. I think it's gotten quieter!"

Emmy's in-session hypnosis and commitment to at-home practice enabled her to achieve a degree of relief she had not known in a decade. She also slept better and was less distressed in general. Shortly afterward, she concluded her sessions of formal hypnosis but continued to practice self-hypnosis as a way to maintain and further her healing.

Misconceptions about Hypnosis

In movies and on TV, hypnotic trance has often been portrayed as a type of "zombified" stupor, where the subject of the trance is lulled into total unconsciousness via a dangling pocket watch or a hypnotist's bug-eyed stare. This is *not* what will happen to you during clinical hypnosis (or any time, for that matter).

Some of the more common misconceptions about hypnosis are:

- That the hypnotherapist controls your mind
- That only unintelligent or weak-willed people can be hypnotized
- That it is a "magic" cure for symptoms
- That you will fall rapidly into a deep trance, after which you will remember nothing about it

What is *actually* true about hypnosis is:

1. All hypnosis is really self-hypnosis. If you are particularly suggestible or unconsciously want someone else to take control, or make decisions for you, you will likely facilitate this happening in one way or another. But the choice of whether you will be hypnotized is yours. Stage hypnotists,

who are *not* clinicians, use hypnotic techniques and also preselect demonstration subjects based on their willingness to comply with the hypnotist's suggestions. If the volunteers enter into trance (and sometimes they may simply be performing to please the hypnotist), it is because they choose to do so.

2. Clinical hypnotherapists—that is, licensed clinicians who are formally trained and certified in clinical hypnosis—adhere to codes of conduct that emphasize their role as collaborators in helping you achieve your healthiest goals. That includes explaining the process of hypnosis clearly, discussing treatment goals with you up front, and supporting you whether or not you decide hypnosis is for you.

3. Most people can enter some level of hypnotic trance, and it is quite easy for most people to enter a light trance (something that happens naturally anyway).

4. Hypnosis is considered a valid and effective treatment for pain, nausea, anxiety, and other issues. But like all other treatments, it does not work for everyone or every condition, nor will it work all of the time.

5. A small percentage of people are able to achieve very deep trances that are so engrossing that they feel similar to sleep. A trance this deep will typically only happen during hypnotherapy with a therapist who is familiar to you, and with whom you feel very comfortable. It will also usually happen only following a long induction period, or if you are fairly tired when you enter into trance. Deep trance states are *not* sleep, however, nor are they necessary for a good outcome. If you enter into a very deep trance state that feels like sleep, you may not consciously remember the specific suggestions after you have re-alerted, but your unconscious mind will have heard them and decided which suggestions to take in for your benefit.

QUESTION

How do I know if I can benefit from hypnosis?
Some important factors that increase the likelihood of success include your natural degree of hypnotizability, how comfortable you feel with both the idea of hypnosis and your therapist, being creative, and being open to new experiences.

In general, whether created spontaneously and indirectly in your normal daily life or as part of hypnotherapy, quite often the trance you achieve will be fairly light, especially if you are new to hypnosis. This will also be the case if you are unsure whether you want to enter trance or prefer to remain more alert to your outer experiences. Furthermore, your mind will not take in hypnotic suggestions that are at odds with what you want or believe is right for you. A well-trained hypnotherapist will also explicitly inform you of this last fact and will give your unconscious mind the suggestion to shape the trance in the way that is for your greatest benefit.

During light trances, you will simply feel relaxed and a bit daydreamy, similar to how you feel while you are washing dishes or preparing a meal but thinking about a party you will attend later in the evening. There will be moments when the images you "see" of who will be at the party will be more prominent for you than the potatoes you are peeling or the plate you are washing, even though you will retain enough attention on the task at hand to continue doing it. If you are in a light or medium-depth trance in a hypnotherapy session, you will still be able to hear and respond verbally to your therapist (if you choose) while noticing the images forming in your mind or the suggestions to feel comfortable, decrease sensations of pain, and increase feelings of comfort.

FACT

In general, you are probably more naturally hypnotizable if you often find yourself getting lost in a book or movie, and tend to be daydreamy. But even those considered "low-hypnotizables" have benefited from hypnosis.

Because most hypnotic trances range from light to medium-deep in that although you are engrossed in your inner world, you retain conscious awareness of your "outer" world—trance will simply feel like the outside world has temporarily moved off to the side of your awareness for the time being. But if you wanted or needed to, you would most likely and quite naturally shift your attention back to whatever is going on outside you. It's actually quite common for people to report feeling that their awareness shifts back and forth from the "movie" in their minds to whatever is going on around them, and back again—whether they are experiencing an everyday or formal trance.

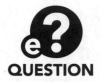

What is a hypnotic induction?
This refers to a technique that helps you enter into a trance state. Examples include counting backward from ten down to one, or fixing your eyes on a spot on the wall, to help you shift to a more daydreamy but focused state.

Naturalistic or Everyday Trances

Trance states are often induced or created via the use of specific imagery, but, technically, no specific imagery is required for hypnosis to occur. For example, if you think back to the last time you were a passenger in a car at night, you may recall becoming much more focused on a memory, daydream, or concern than on the blur of trees or other scenery rushing past the window as you sped down the highway.

If you were the driver, you probably noticed that at certain times you were more focused on the traffic in front of you or were actively keeping an eye out for your exit. At other times, more of your awareness may have been on having an imagined conversation with someone or thinking about what you needed from the grocery store, or "working" on a project for your job—even though your body remained in the car and your eyes were focused on the road the entire time. The monotony of viewing the yellow center line on a roadway, the hum of the car's engine, and fatigue all are trance inducing. Again, anything rhythmic or repetitive can induce a trance, and if you are tired, you may notice feeling "trance-y" more readily.

Guided Imagery

Guided imagery involves the deliberate, "guided" shaping of your mind's experience of an inner journey. Although the term "imagery" usually calls to mind the use of the visual sense, the most effective imagery tends to mimic what your brain does naturally when you daydream, and thus creates an experience that is multisensory. The "guide" in guided imagery can be the voice of your therapist, leading you through an in-session imaginal "journey" such as through a tropical rainforest; across a warm, sandy beach; or to another place of comfort. The multisensory language used to shape this exercise may include feeling the warmth and grittiness of the sand against your bare feet, the smell of the sea air, the sound of waves crashing along the shoreline, and perhaps an inner sense of profound peace.

Imagery can also be primarily emotional or even feeling-oriented in nature. As an example, you might focus your attention on the remembered sensation of comfort in an area of your body that has been in pain. You might also recall a time when you felt particularly calm and notice how you experience this pleasant feeling inside you via relaxed muscles, a sense of safety, and the like.

The Evidence for Imagery

A number of studies have found guided imagery to help decrease symptom severity. Guided imagery has been shown to reduce anticipatory nausea during chemotherapy, decrease anxiety, reduce blood pressure in those with hypertension, reduce postoperative pain, help with fibromyalgia pain, improve adherence to self-care regimens in diabetes, reduce cigarette cravings and smoking, improve sleep, and more.

Imagery has many health benefits that overlap with those associated with other mind-body therapies, such as meditation. Unlike meditation, however, you may find yourself paying attention to the imagery with less effort than that required when focusing on the breath, as imagery is naturally engaging. The most effective and appealing imagery typically engages all the senses rather than just one, such as visual imagery.

FACT

You can enhance the effect of guided imagery by also engaging some of your "actual" senses via pleasant aromas or by incorporating your favorite music or nature sounds recordings. Many guided imagery programs are already set to music designed to further induce relaxation.

How to Find a Qualified Professional

For all the reasons stated previously, it's worth finding a hypnotherapist who is certified by a reputable credentialing organization and as such is licensed in his primary profession, whether this is medicine, psychology, dentistry, etc. Certified clinical hypnotherapists will also maintain membership in the professional associations relevant to their fields, such as the American Medical Association or the American Psychological Association.

Two reputable hypnosis-accrediting organizations are the American Society of Clinical Hypnosis (ASCH; *www.ASCH.net*) and the Society for Clinical and Experimental Hypnosis (SCEH; *www.sceh.us*). Each maintains a list of providers they have certified.

With regard to guided imagery, there is no formal training requirement. Many cognitive-behavioral and other therapists use imagery as part of their work, and other health professionals may either deliver guided imagery to help you relax prior to or during a medical or dental procedure, or make prerecorded programs available for your use. It's worth asking your current or any prospective providers if they use imagery in their work with patients.

When Hypnotic Imagery Goes Awry

Guided imagery and hypnosis are safe and effective practices for achieving healthy goals, including that of pain management. As mentioned earlier in the chapter, however, everyone creates their own imagery all the time, even without thinking about it. This includes not only the things you wish for, enjoy, or are healthy for you but also, quite often your mind fixates very intently on what you dislike, what causes you distress, and what you are worried about. You will probably notice this is especially true when your pain is high, and when you feel anxious, fearful, depressed, or angry. In fact, when you catastrophize or come to the most catastrophic, awful conclusion about your pain (e.g., "This is terrible! I will never be able to handle this!"), your mind is quite probably forming very intense images of all the worst possible situations or outcomes associated with your distress.

It's especially important to become aware of the negative imagery you create, even if it's understandable given what you are going through. Otherwise, and in addition to further worsening your mood, you may inadvertently create the bodily experience that you fear. This was illustrated in a 2004 study conducted by researchers at the University of Pittsburgh Medical Center of people whose pain was induced in the laboratory. As expected, experiencing physical pain caused changes in brain activity and also led to self-reports of moderate-level pain. What was novel about this study was that hypnotic suggestions to feel pain *also* caused changes in brain activity, and participants reported feeling pain as a result—albeit less intensely—even though nothing was done to cause physical pain.

It's worth noting that in this study, participants were also asked to simply imagine being in pain, but were not given hypnotic suggestions to this effect. Although imagining being in pain did not result in self-reported pain, it also, to an even lesser extent, impacted brain activity as if they were in pain.

In 2009, the same researchers, now at the University of Birmingham in the United Kingdom, used fMRI to examine the effects of suggestions on increasing or decreasing pain in patients diagnosed with fibromyalgia. Specifically, the team examined the effects of suggestions both following and without prior hypnotic induction. They found that both with and without hypnotic induction, suggestions to change pain severity resulted in observable changes in brain activity in a number of areas. Participants reported feeling they had more control over pain severity if they had been hypnotized, however. Furthermore, the observed magnitude of change in brain activity was greater in several areas of the brain following a formal hypnotic induction. Therefore, the type of imagery you generate, or trance you find yourself in, can have a very real effect on your brain and your experience of pain.

The takeaway from these findings is *not* that you must completely block out any thoughts of pain, but that it's worth becoming more aware of the imagery you tend to create when stressed or uncomfortable. Your brain is a very powerful tool, and with some practice you can use imagery or self-hypnosis for easing pain and increasing calm, rather than inadvertently worsening pain symptoms.

Who Should Not Use Imagery or Hypnosis?

If any of the following apply to you, you should seek the counsel of a licensed mental health professional who is certified in clinical hypnotherapy before using at-home imagery or hypnosis programs:

- If your anxiety or depression have been longstanding or severe
- If you have thoughts of hurting yourself (or others)
- If you have times when you feel disconnected from reality, or if you have been diagnosed with a severe mental illness such as a psychotic illness
- If your ability to cope is compromised to the point where your daily functioning is impaired
- If you have tried an at-home guided imagery or hypnosis audio and noticed an increase in your mood or pain symptoms
- If you have tried hypnosis with a professional and noticed a worsening of symptoms

Again, for the majority of people, imagery and hypnosis are generally very safe tools that you "use" anyway—just by virtue of having a mind. Most people can use the imagery and hypnosis audio programs developed by health professionals, as these should be carefully designed to maximize calm and comfort.

There are a number of companies that sell imagery and hypnosis audio programs to foster relaxation and pain relief. The two most well known are probably HealthJourneys.com and SoundsTrue.com. You can also create and record your own imagery and even set it to your favorite music or nature sounds for relaxing. One resource for free nature sounds is *http://meditationroom.org*. One ocean wave track in particular pairs especially well with hypnotic imagery. You can access this track here: *http://meditationroom.org/free-nature-sounds/ocean-waves-audio/*.

Hypnotic Imagery Script for Pain Relief

This script incorporates hypnotic imagery and suggestions to reduce emotional distress and enhance physical comfort. You'll notice that the structure of hypnotic language is different from the way you might normally word things, in order to let your "daytime," logical mind take a well-deserved vacation. You will also notice that the word "pain" is not used, to keep the emphasis on fostering feelings of calm, well-being, and ease—the opposite of pain. This type of wording will help you achieve a trance state that can help you take in the suggestions at a deeper level, and give your body permission to get as comfortable as possible.

You may find that you enjoy listening before you go to bed, or when you can set aside a quiet half-hour for yourself. Record in your own voice, or ask someone you know to do so. Feel free to adapt the wording to your liking. Then, make time to listen regularly as part of your self-care program. As with most therapies, you will find increased benefits with practice. Note that the ellipses (. . .) indicate longer pauses. Experiment with the pacing that feels most relaxing for you.

So now, let's begin by observing your breath . . . not trying to change it in any way, but simply noticing . . . the rise of your chest, and the expansion of your belly . . . with each inhalation . . . and the fall of the belly, and relaxation of the chest with each exhalation . . . as if you were standing on the shoreline, simply noticing ocean waves rolling in . . . and out . . . with each in-breath . . . clearing your mind . . . and with each out-breath . . . releasing anything you'd like to release . . . no need to make anything happen . . . relaxation naturally follows the breath . . . and you can notice how as you allow yourself to get really comfortable . . . whatever that is for you in this moment, you can sense with pleasure and appreciation as your muscles gently unwind . . . perhaps becoming aware of the space between your shoulder blades widening . . . your shoulders dropping a little lower . . . your breathing naturally slowing down . . . as you become more comfortable . . . feeling a sense of ease as you settle in to the chair . . . or bed . . . or couch . . . feeling its effortless support . . . such a wonderful thing, to make time for well-being. . . .

And as you relax . . . and release . . . and breathe . . . exactly what you should be doing right now . . . doing the work of letting . . . you can allow any other thoughts or things on your "to do" list to fade off into the distance for now . . . and isn't that such a terrific thing . . . to remember that you can become even more comfortable, simply by observing . . . and letting . . . and releasing. . . . And as you just allow yourself to observe your own body . . . as if you were observing a cloud in the sky . . . with an easy detachment, you may be pleasantly surprised to notice how any discomfort, or any distress, moves off to the side . . . into the background . . . as your awareness of what is comfortable within you . . . something simple, such as the tip of your nose, or perhaps an earlobe, a fingertip . . . it really doesn't matter . . . your mind instinctively moves to whatever is most comfortable for you . . . and so anything else just fades into the periphery . . . no need to try to do anything about it . . . you can simply breathe through any thoughts or feelings or sensations

. . . sending them out to sea with the breath . . . seeing how nice that is . . . and how that naturally turns down the volume on whatever has been too loud . . . creating space between you and whatever has been bothersome . . . until now . . . because now you know that you can expand feelings of comfort . . . and ease . . . breathing them in . . . and delight in how this allows anything else to move off to the side for the time being . . . whatever time is most helpful for you.

And now you can delight as your very wise mind . . . your truest ally and oldest friend . . . a trusted companion who is ready to help you now that you are ready . . . you can enjoy as your mind helps you use your breath to amplify those feelings of comfort and ease and move them to any area of your body or mind that has felt anything other than comfortable. Like water, a sense of ease flows to any areas of tension . . . bringing calm . . . and comfort . . . a release and profound peace. So just stay with these feelings of well-being . . . and breathe. . . . Wonderful. . . . [longer pause—make this as long as you like, even for several minutes].

Allow yourself to sit remaining calm and peacefully focused on your breath for as long as you like . . . and when you are ready, at exactly the right time for you, and in exactly the right way, you can slowly begin to bring your awareness back to the room . . . the ambient sounds . . . noticing the urges to gently stretch and shift as needed . . . and you can slowly open your eyes, taking a few cleansing breaths . . . and you are ready to return to your day.

CHAPTER 11

Mindfulness and the Gift of the Present

Modern life is replete with challenges to living in the present. Among these are things you enjoy, such as watching TV and other distractions, as well as things that are decidedly unpleasant, such as chronic pain. When you are bored, feel unwell, are anxious about something, or feel impatient for the future to come, you likely move your attention out of the present moment. Yet the here-and-now is the only time you will ever truly experience your life. It is the only time you ever have. *Period*. And it is also where all change occurs, including change that can calm your mind and ease your body. So it is worth learning how to be in the moment.

The Practice of Mindfulness

Mindfulness, also known as insight meditation, is most simply described as "present-moment, nonjudgmental awareness." It is a practice that, although derived from Buddhist tradition, in essence is simply the active attention to and acceptance of the present moment, whatever that happens to be.

Mindfulness is referred to as a "practice" because it requires your conscious decision and effort to be aware and attentive in this particular way. There are two basic ways of engaging in mindfulness practice. The first is via focused attention. Focused attention involves deliberately attending to a neutral point of awareness, such as the sensations and rhythm of your own breathing.

FACT

Many people get caught up in "liking" or "not liking" what they observe, especially during boring, unpleasant, or uncomfortable experiences, like waiting in line. Yet, liking or not liking is similar to any other type of mental event—simply observe, describe, and return your awareness to the present.

The "How" of Mindfulness

Normally, you breathe day and night, rarely noticing the depth, rate, or quality of your breath, or the sensation of air entering your nostrils, filling your lungs, and expanding your abdomen. Mindfulness practice encourages you to observe whenever the mind starts to wander (which it inevitably will). In fact, your mind will likely have many thoughts about the experience of observing your breath (e.g., "Why am I doing this?" or "How is this supposed to help?" or "I'm bored.").

Your mind will also almost certainly drift off to mental events that are more engaging or entertaining, such as pleasant memories, daydreams, things you wish for, and the like. If you are anxious or depressed, or if your pain is high, however, your mind will probably drift to negative events or feelings about the past, your emotional assessment of physical discomfort, or your worries or fears about the future. You may also become aware of judgments about the process ("This is silly; breathing isn't going to change anything for me!")

or perhaps judgments about your mindfulness "performance" ("I can't even master this breathing thing properly! I'm just not doing it right.").

In fact, your mind is just doing what it typically does; leap-frogging from one thought or feeling to another . . . and another . . . and another, until you are several lily pads away from the experience of observing your breath.

And that is a completely normal part of the process of learning to focus your attention. As you notice these thoughts, feelings, memories, judgments, or physical sensations, the key is to *observe*, *describe*, and *move your attention* once again back to observing your breath—even if you have to do this a thousand times. Because engaging in this process has been shown to increase the thickness of the frontal areas of your brain (a good thing!), which in turn will make it easier to remain calm, be focused, and better manage your pain.

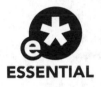

ESSENTIAL

You may find, especially when starting out, that your mindfulness practice benefits from some form of structure or guidance. Dr. Jon Kabat-Zinn has produced several instructional CDs, which are available from his website: *www.mindfulnesscds.com*. There are also a number of free mindfulness downloads available, such as these through UCLA: *http://marc.ucla.edu.*

When you are beginning a mindfulness practice, you may feel that sometimes it seems much easier to remain focused on your breath than at other times. It's normal to question your ability to be mindful, or to become frustrated with your progress. Remember that these thoughts and feelings are simply mental events, and you can incorporate noticing them into your practice. It's also worth keeping in mind these four keys to engaging in mindful awareness:

1. *Observe.* Notice what you notice—your rate, rhythm, and sensations of your breath. Simply observe the thoughts or emotions, physical sensations, or judgments when they move across your mental screen.
2. *Describe.* When you become aware of something other than your breath—a thought, emotion, judgment, memory, association, or physical

sensation—moving across your mental screen, notice and then describe it (e.g., "There is a thought about my shopping list," "There is a judgment that this is a silly practice," or "There is the sensation of cramping in my back.").

3. *Return.* You have thus far duly noted the mental event or physical sensation and described it. Now, bring your awareness back once again to observing the rate, rhythm, quality, etc., of your breathing, as many times as necessary.

4. *Breathe.* Use your breath to help you "breathe through" any distractions, and shift your awareness back to your inhalation and exhalation.

Mindfulness Exercise

To develop a mindfulness practice involves setting aside a regular time each day, just as you would schedule or prioritize any other important commitment. In the beginning, you may wish to set aside five minutes in the morning or in the evening before you go to bed. Set a timer if you like, so you can release any worries about finishing "on schedule." Feel free to record the following instructions to guide your practice initially.

Allow your awareness, like a flashlight beam in a dim room, to reveal, highlight, or focus on your breath. Again, notice the air as it moves in through your nostrils, being aware of the physical sensations, whether the temperature, or "texture," the sound of your breath, the feeling of your chest and abdomen expanding gently with each inhalation . . . noticing the pause at the top of the inhalation, and then observing as the breath moves back out through your nose, passing your nostrils . . . your belly and chest gently relaxing back down as you exhale . . . the natural pause before you inhale once again. When thoughts, feelings, judgments, or physical sensations move across your mind, as they invariably will, just observe them as you would any other event. Say to yourself, "there is a thought of my to-do list," or "there is a sensation of tightness in my hip flexors," or there is the judgment, "this is silly." Whatever it is that you notice, simply breathe. . . . Bring your awareness again back to observing your breath moving in . . . and out . . . as if you were observing ocean waves moving back and forth . . . or clouds moving effortlessly across the sky. Breathe.

Finish your session by attending to your breath for however long you have decided to practice today. Over time, gradually increase your practice to ten minutes, then fifteen, then twenty. Practice for longer if you like. Enjoy the feelings of calm and stillness that mindfulness will foster.

Open Monitoring

The second style of mindfulness meditation that you may hear or read about is referred to as open monitoring. Open monitoring is also referred to as "choiceless awareness." With open monitoring, rather than anchoring the attention on the breath, one receptively notices whatever comes into one's field of awareness, almost as if you were standing at a window and simply observing whatever crossed in front of it—a car driving down the street, a family walking slowly by, a jogger racing past, a dog walker with his charges barking as they pass your home. You could only observe these while they were in the frame of the window, and then you would notice what passed by next, and so forth. Again, the aim is to notice without attaching to any individual thoughts, feelings, or physical sensations.

This practice can further help you become aware of and free yourself from your mental and emotional habits and whatever types of inner experiences tend to derail you in some way. Open monitoring is considered a more advanced type of practice, and you may find that you benefit from seeking formal guidance via a meditation teacher or class, or via an audio recording.

Why Be in the Present?

If you are in pain, you almost certainly have thought, "I'd rather be almost *anywhere* than in the present," and yet there are a number of reasons why it is worth cultivating the ability to be where you are, so to speak.

The first is that the present moment is the only one you will ever have. Period. The past that you mentally revisit or rehash is done. And while the past was occurring, it *was* the present moment. Each time you remember it, the past will be experienced slightly differently, with some new layer or interpretation or wish overlaid onto it.

The future that you hope will be easier for you, or fear will be too challenging, will undoubtedly be at least somewhat different, if not quite a bit different, from however you imagine it now. And when the future arrives, *it will be the present.*

Perhaps most important, the present moment is where all change happens. You learn from the past and plan for the future, in the present. You make moment-to-moment decisions to keep things the same (sometimes simply by choosing not to do anything differently), or perhaps you take an active role in making a different choice from the one you might usually make. But, again, in the present moment you keep things the same, or perhaps decide to take action, and these choices are what shape your life. In essence, what happens in the now is akin to the brick you use to pave the road ahead or build the foundation of your life.

Oscar and the "Angry Walk"

When Oscar decided to go to therapy, his body was the only thing he felt he could control. An extremely disciplined and competitive young man, he was constantly pushing himself to become stronger, faster, and do more. When Oscar fractured a bone in his foot, he prided himself on "toughing out the pain" and continuing to run, despite his doctor's recommendation to stay off his feet. Oscar believed that if he kept his body strong enough, he would always be "okay." Yet, Oscar struggled with anxiety and the belief that he was *not okay* unless he was achieving something. He also felt frequent frustration with friends, coworkers, and family members whom he thought should be as achievement-oriented and "tough" as he was. Oscar admitted he was also constantly in a hurry and could not understand why anyone would slow down—ever. Even strangers on the street annoyed Oscar to no end.

"When I'm walking to work in the morning, it's like these people are moving so slowly—like they have nowhere to be! What the heck is wrong with them?"

Although Oscar was fairly critical of others, he also worried that they either did not understand or didn't like him. Oscar reported having frequent insomnia, waking in the middle of the night worrying about work, obsessing over what people thought of him, and the like.

When the topic of mindfulness came up, Oscar worried he was too "type A" to meditate. When he learned that mindfulness could help calm his anxiety, feel less frustrated, and improve his sleep, however, he agreed to give it a try. Initially, Oscar practiced observing his breath for two minutes every morning, and soon after began noticing subtle benefits. The feelings of calm he noticed led him to increase the length of his practice to five minutes, and then ten minutes. After a few months, Oscar further increased his "quiet time" to twenty minutes each morning, adding one-minute "mini-sessions" whenever he felt particularly stressed at work.

"I love this technique! I can be in a meeting, with people getting stressed all around me, and I can bring my focus to my breath for a minute—no one notices I'm doing this." Oscar smiled proudly. "But lots of people have noticed how much more relaxed I am. And get this—I was walking to work the other day, and there were all of the people ahead of me, doing that 'slow-poke' thing that I usually can't stand. My first thought was, 'I'm going to blow these people off the line, so to speak,' and I started to speed up to pass them. And then I realized that, 'Hey, I have plenty of time before I have to be at work. I could simply walk and just notice whatever is around me—the people, the trees, the sound of my feet connecting with the sidewalk.' And then all of a sudden, I wasn't doing my usual 'angry walk' anymore. I was simply walking."

Oscar's anxiety and frustration had ceased to dominate his body-mind. He also worried less and less about whether he was "performing" well enough for people to like him and, instead, allowed himself to just "be." He reported sleeping better, having better interactions with loved ones and strangers alike, and overall feeling happier.

How Mindfulness Might Change You

Although becoming more aware of living in the present moment seems like a purely mental experience, mindfulness has been shown to have benefits far beyond subjective changes in awareness (not to discount these!). At a minimum, you will probably notice feeling calmer and less reactive in general. You will likely also feel less reactive to situations, people, thoughts, and physical sensations that used to leave you feeling sad, angry, worried, or frustrated. Your sleep should improve. Your memory of life experiences, from the mundane (e.g., walking your child to school, reaching an exercise goal) to the sublime (e.g., watching your child take his first steps, seeing your child graduate high school, knowing that someone loves you, achieving something important to you) will be enhanced—because you will actually have "been there" for these moments.

In addition, you will likely become even more skilled at determining when a bodily sensation is a normal variation or response to something (such as your stomach hurting because you ate an unfamiliar food, or muscles aching because you slept in a different position or tried a new exercise) versus when they are a cause for alarm. Being able to make this type of distinction should significantly decrease your anxiety about your health and help you feel better in general.

Mindfulness can be paired with any of the other treatments mentioned in this book to help you become more present, calmer, make better choices, and feel more comfortable in your own body. CBT, hypnosis, aromatherapy, massage, exercise, and healthy eating are some examples.

With regard to mood, you may very well notice that symptoms of general anxiety, depression, or anger release much of their hold on you because the worried, angry, or hopeless thoughts will become mental events that you can observe without automatically identifying with them or taking them as true.

Health Benefits of Mindfulness

Dr. Jon Kabat-Zinn, a Massachusetts Institute of Technology-trained molecular biologist, is frequently credited with bringing the concept and practice of mindfulness to the Western medical community. In the late 1980s and early 1990s, Dr. Kabat-Zinn was at the University of Massachusetts Medical Center and began teaching Mindfulness-Based Stress Reduction (MBSR) to medically ill patients, including those in chronic pain. What Dr. Kabat-Zinn and other colleagues found is that an eight-week program emphasizing mindfulness via breath awareness, gentle yoga, a technique called the body scan, and other exercises helped patients significantly decrease distress, increase calm, decrease pain severity, and improve pain coping. Since the program's creation, thousands of people have completed MBSR programs, and many, many others have learned to use simple techniques to foster greater mindfulness in daily life.

In addition to easing the sensation of pain and improving coping, mindfulness fosters a state of relaxation that can be more restorative than sleep, and in fact has been shown to facilitate sleep in people who suffer from insomnia. Mindfulness practice lowers levels of stress hormones and can increase the levels of brain chemicals associated with positive mood (such as serotonin).

Furthermore, mindfulness practice is associated with improved immune functioning, enhanced working (immediate) memory, improved relationships, and decreased rumination (the tendency to focus on negative thoughts, feelings, and memories). Mindfulness has also been found to help in the treatment of eating disorders, and to improve coping and quality of life in those with serious medical diagnoses.

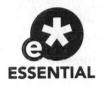

ESSENTIAL

If you are taking medication as part of your pain management plan, it's vital to remember to take it on schedule and at the correct dose. Learning to become more aware in the present can help you better remember when and how much of your medication to take.

Mindfulness for Chronic Pain

Chronic pain and its associated distress activate the "fight or flight" response—the same response that would occur if you were under threat of attack by another person or wild animal, or faced some other form of imminent danger. In fact, your body and mind respond to *internal* threats—stressful thoughts or physical sensations—the way they respond to *external* threats (e.g., a bear in the woods or someone chasing you). Your heart rate, blood pressure, muscle tension, blood sugar, and stress hormones all increase in response to any perceived threat, regardless of whether you decide to stay and fight, or attempt to flee the scene.

Of course, with the stressor chronic pain, there really isn't an effective way to "flee." Common ways people try to flee the experience of pain include sleeping too much, overeating, drinking alcohol, and overusing prescription or street drugs. Having chronic pain lowers the "pain threshold," meaning that it will take less physical stimulation to trigger the sensation of pain. And the more apprehensive or distressed you are about pain, the more likely it is that your pain will feel more severe and less bearable, and that you will castastrophize about your ability to tolerate pain or live a meaningful life despite pain. Catastrophizing will perpetuate and worsen the pain experience overall and compromise your quality of life.

The good news is that research on mindfulness, in addition to showing that it reduces reactivity to stress and increases calm and well-being, also improves pain coping and decreases pain severity. You may also find yourself relying less on medications and other substances, such as alcohol, to quiet your pain.

Mindfulness and the Brain

Using special imaging techniques to view brain activity and thickness, researchers discovered that people who have practiced mindfulness meditation for some time have increased thickness in several brain areas—notably, in parts of the brain associated with paying attention, remaining calm, and managing pain. Mindfulness also seems to "rewire" the brain such that some areas tend to become more active, and thus better able to reframe the experience of pain, while other areas become less active, thereby allowing meditators to be less emotionally reactive to pain. These findings are considered particularly important because they show that mindfulness results in observable physical and functional brain changes that have a very real, positive, and measurable impact on the pain experience.

QUESTION

I've heard mindfulness can help my depression—is this true?
Yes! In fact, Mindfulness-Based Cognitive Therapy (MBCT) is as effective as antidepressants in preventing depression relapse after a successful treatment. MBCT can be combined with antidepressants, and for some people can be used on its own.

Mindfulness and Aging

Another groundbreaking line of research has shown that mindfulness practice blunts the physical effects of stress by lengthening telomeres, which are "caps" at the end of chromosomes. (Chromosomes are strands of DNA that contain genes.) Dr. Elizabeth Blackburn, a Nobel prize-winning researcher, has likened telomeres to the plastic caps on the ends of shoelaces that prevent them from fraying. She and Dr. Elissa Epel, a Yale-educated health psychologist, have engaged in a number of studies on the impact of stress and lifestyle factors on telomere length. Dr. Blackburn's research was the first to establish the link between shorter telomeres and having a shorter lifespan.

In general, telomeres shorten with age. Shorter telomeres are also found in people with diabetes, heart disease, osteoarthritis, Alzheimer's, and other illnesses, regardless of age. Blackburn and Epel found that chronic stress, such as that found in mothers caring for chronically ill children, or in those caring for a chronically ill partner, was associated with shorter telomeres, and thus greater risk of premature aging and illness. The researchers believe that when the brain appraises a situation as threatening, and dwells on the negatives associated with this situation, this keeps the body in a prolonged state of fight-or-flight. Again, that state is useful if you need to flee from an attacker, but becomes harmful to the body and mind if experienced for an extended period of time.

What Drs. Epel and Blackburn's research has found preliminarily is that mindfulness meditation helps the brain decrease rumination and reframe stressful events as "challenges" rather than inevitable threats. A challenge is something you can work to overcome, as opposed to a threat you need to "escape" from or "knock out" (neither of which is appropriate when dealing with chronic illness, even if you are "fighting" to manage symptoms). Reframing threats as challenges and decreasing rumination not only helps you feel better emotionally, but also is beneficial for your body—even at the cellular level. Mindfulness is also linked to more positive mood in general. Furthermore, mindfulness helps foster acceptance of those things that cannot be avoided or changed. All of these benefits help prevent premature aging and illness.

Acceptance and Pain

Mindfulness, in contrast to the experience of pain, tends to generate a state of peace, increased calm, and acceptance. Many people confuse the concept of acceptance with resignation and avoidance, but there are important differences between these states. Acceptance implies a willingness or ability to be with the situation as it is, rather than resisting what cannot be changed. Resisting something you can't alter is futile and exhausting. Giving up and avoiding the situation or idea altogether is also unproductive and prevents you experiencing the life you actually have, even if it is not exactly as you would ideally want it to be. And as you have probably noticed, resisting or fighting feelings of pain, or attempting to flee from them are both ineffective ways of managing pain. The pain and distress remain.

Acceptance, in contrast, has been shown to improve pain coping and has been linked to reduced anxiety and depression, reduced pain severity, reduced disability, and improved physical and psychological functioning overall. Acceptance also frees you up to do what you can to improve your situation when this is possible, without dwelling on what you cannot do.

Everyday, Informal Mindfulness Practice

As described in the previous sections, the traditionally taught way of practicing mindfulness is to set aside a regular time each day to attend to your breath, notice the thoughts, feelings, and judgments that naturally arise, and once again bring your awareness to your breath, observing it as if you were observing any other activity, object, or process. There are many ways to be mindful, however, and the simple decision to be present during normal daily activities will also enhance calm and focus, decrease distress, and enhance your ability to live a life you can appreciate and enjoy, despite pain. You will find that things you previously found boring or tedious, such as waiting in line, doing laundry, or being stuck in traffic, will become opportunities to be present, aware, and peaceful.

Here are some examples of ways to practice everyday mindfulness:

- *Washing the dishes.* Notice the temperature of the water against your hands, whether you wear gloves or not. Observe the sounds of the water running, the dishes clanking against flatware, the play of light across soap bubbles. Take in the aroma of the dish detergent. Feel the weight of a dish, a glass, or a fork in your hands.
- *Walking.* Notice the rhythm of your walk, the sound of your footsteps on the floor or pavement. Become aware of the impulse to move one foot,

raise a knee, step forward, or stop at a street corner. Take in the sights, sounds, and scents in your environment.

- *Showering.* Hear the water flowing out of the showerhead and onto your skin, notice the sound it makes when it connects with the shower floor or wall or door. Feel the pressure of the spray on your face, your back, your arms, your feet, and notice the temperature of the water. Feel the weight of the bar of soap, the bottle of shampoo, and notice the sudsiness of the lather. Become aware of the different aromas of your soap, shampoo, shaving cream, even if these are "unscented." Notice as your mind wanders to thoughts of the day, or the past, or the future, and bring your attention once again back to the shower experience.

- *Eating.* Notice the thoughts that lead you to choose to eat one food over another. Become aware of your body's readiness to eat, such as your stomach growling or your mouth watering. Take in your food first with your eyes, then your nose. Hear the sound of your fork piercing a vegetable and then your teeth chewing your food, making it increasingly smooth and easier to digest with each movement of your teeth and tongue against whatever you are chewing. Observe the texture and taste of your food as it moves through your lips, between your teeth. Notice the impulse to swallow, and perhaps follow a bite with a sip of water. Try to observe when you begin to feel satisfied and how this is different from the sensations of feeling hungry or full.

- *Talking.* When you enter into conversation with someone, notice the difference between actively listening versus thinking ahead to your response. Become aware of the other person's facial expressions, tone, and pauses. Observe the impulse to interrupt, or contradict, or agree. Give yourself time and space to formulate your thoughts, choose your words, or simply listen. Notice what you later remember about the conversation when you actively listen versus when your mind wanders. Be aware of your emotional reactions, judgments, or thoughts as you listen and speak.

- *Sleeping.* Become aware of your body's signals that it is time for bed. Notice the scent of your bedding, the temperature of your bedroom, and any ambient sounds. Observe the texture of your sheets, comforter, or blanket, the softness or firmness of your pillows. If you have a partner, notice the sounds of her breathing, the warmth of his body near yours. Observe and breathe through any thoughts, such as "I only have five more hours of sleep left," or "Tomorrow I will have to give a presentation." Attend to the sounds of your own breathing, the rise and fall of your chest and abdomen, the comfortable pressure of your hands resting on your belly.

The Practice of Loving Kindness

Also referred to as "Metta," the practice of loving kindness is an aspect of mindfulness practice that can help you increase contentment and compassion, develop greater love for yourself and others, and foster forgiveness. Loving kindness can also help you develop a sense of connection to all beings, without exception. It is a practice that can be uniquely healing and freeing because it allows you to release negative emotional ties to those with whom you have had some sort of discord, who have wronged you, or disappointed you—including when that person has been you, yourself.

You may find that at first it seems especially challenging to send loving kindness to people you have strong negative feelings about, and that's perfectly fine. Just notice whenever feelings arise and breathe through them. Over time, the practice will feel more and more natural, and very freeing.

Loving Kindness Exercise

Begin by finding a time and place where you can devote a few minutes to the practice that follows. Sit comfortably and simply observe your breathing for a few breaths. Imagine the breath moving in and out of your heart. Be with this feeling. Say to yourself, silently, "May I be happy. May I be well. May I be safe. May I be peaceful and at ease."

Allow yourself to take in each statement at a deep level. Notice how you feel as you do so. Breathe.

Next, recall someone for whom you care deeply or who has cared for you. Hold the image of them in your mind. Repeat these phrases of loving kindness toward them: "May you be happy. May you be well. May you be safe. May you be peaceful and at ease." Again, notice how it feels to send loving kindness, this time to another. Breathe.

Now, you can direct loving kindness to other specific people, animals, and all beings. Note those who come to mind. Repeat these phrases to each one, breathing in feelings of love and peace, and breathing through or simply observing difficult emotions or thoughts. Notice how this feels, and how your emotions and judgments can shift over time—even during the same session.

You can conclude your practice by saying, "May all beings be happy. May all beings be well. May all beings be safe. May all beings be peaceful and at ease."

Quite a bit has been written about loving kindness, and there are many variations with regard to wording. Create the phrasing that feels most right to you. To learn more, you may wish to read works by renowned teachers such as Jack Kornfield, Sharon Salzberg, or Tara Brach. You can listen to free loving kindness and other mindfulness meditations on Tara Brach's website: *www.tarabrach.com*.

A 2008 study with 139 adults found that the practice of loving kindness increased positive emotions such as love, joy, gratitude, contentment, and hope, and was also associated with mindful attention, self-acceptance, positive relations with others, enhanced quality of life, and better physical health. To access the research article, visit: *www.ncbi.nlm.nih.gov/pmc/articles/PMC3156028/*.

There's an App for That

There are a number of low-cost apps that can help you begin and maintain a mindfulness practice:

- *Simply Being* is a popular app available for IOS and Android that provides step-by-step mindfulness instruction and allows you to set a time for five, ten, fifteen, or twenty minutes. You can listen to the exercise with or without music or nature sounds in the background. For more information, visit *www.meditationoasis.com*.
- *Headspace* is another popular app that offers a free ten-day meditation training feature that promises to teach the basics of mindfulness in ten, ten-minute sessions. After that, you can subscribe to access more

content that is tailored to particular needs, situations, and timeframes. You can also connect with your friends who use the app. Visit *www .headspace.com/headspace-meditation-app* for more information.

- *Insight Timer* is yet another app available for free for iOS and Android. The app guides your mindfulness practice with the soothing sounds of Tibetan bowls to begin and end your meditation. You can see how many people around the world, and in which locations, are currently meditating using the app at any given time. This app also allows you to connect with other meditators, track your progress, save various meditation routines, and more. Visit *https://insighttimer.com* to learn more or download.

CHAPTER 12

Energy Therapies

There are many different terms for energy, such as qi, chi, and prana. Energy healing represents a range of approaches, from movement therapies (covered in Chapter 7), including Qigong, tai chi, and yoga, to healing systems like Reiki. Acupuncture (covered in Chapter 14) purports to move and balance chi through the placement of fine needles. Even homeopathic therapies fall under the energy medicine umbrella because they are extremely dilute, and in many cases are thought only to contain the energetic imprint of the active substances.

A Benign but Controversial Category

Some systems of healing, such as acupuncture and laying-on of hands, have been around for thousands of years. Throughout the ages, people have engaged in one form or another of trying to channel the divine or create balance by affecting the life force of those who are ill.

Other approaches, such as movement therapies, in addition to being ancient in origin can put the person doing them squarely in the driver's seat—you either decide to practice Qigong, tai chi, or yoga, or you don't. (A form of Qigong referred to as external Qigong involves a practitioner moving someone else's qi, but that is outside the scope of this chapter.)

Is Qi the Key?

Exercises that supposedly shift one's energy have particular appeal for those who like to be active participants in achieving and maintaining health. As mentioned previously, yoga, tai chi, and Qigong are linked to a number of health benefits. Whether these benefits are due solely to the effects of physical training and enhanced relaxation, or whether the energetic component adds something additional has not been definitively concluded according to modern scientific methods. Therefore, the answer to what is the "magic ingredient" in these therapies may never be known for certain. Most people who engage in some sort of gentle movement on a regular basis wind up feeling better regardless of whether there is an energetic component to the practice. Yet, proponents would assert that there is a difference between physical disciplines that balance qi and other forms of exercise.

Challenges to Evaluating Energy Therapies

NASA physicist-turned-energy healer Barbara Brennan has said that the energy field is made up of multiple layers, or levels, each one penetrating the body's tissues and together extending several inches beyond the skin. There is debate in the scientific community about whether there is an energy field at all, however, as it is considered undetectable by most people. In addition, a 1998 study published in the *Journal of the American Medical Association (JAMA)* found that energy healers were unable to detect the presence versus the absence of the human energy field. The study was widely publicized as proof that there was no validity to energy healing.

The JAMA study just mentioned was authored by Emily Rosa, then a nine-year-old girl who, with her mother, conducted the experiment for Emily's science fair project. You can read the full research article here: *http://jama.jamanetwork.com/article.aspx?articleid=187390.*

The Rosa family's findings were in contrast to those of Dr. Gary Schwartz, formerly of Yale University and now at the University of Arizona. Together with his colleagues, Dr. Schwartz has conducted several studies related to energy healing. Data from some of his studies found that many people can, in fact, sense the biofield, or human energy field. Dr. Schwartz's work has also found that energy healing was linked to enhanced well being in humans, decreases in heart rate in animals who were exposed to a stressor, and that Reiki was protective against noise-induced microvascular (small blood vessel) leakage in rats.

A 2004 study by Dr. Schwartz and colleagues found that both music and energy healing significantly increased the number of zucchini and okra seeds that germinated within a 72 hour period as compared to seeds in the control conditions. Details about Dr. Schwartz's research can be found in his book, *The Energy Healing Experiments.*

Hands-on healing helps the receiver feel cared for and comforted. In a day and age where an increasing number of relationships or communications are "virtual," many people are left craving attention from a caring presence or a compassionate touch. Because of this fact, visiting *any* attentive provider—CAM or conventional—can feel healing. And positive emotions on their own have been associated with better mental and physical health and improved quality of life.

This information is not mentioned to take away from any *actual* effect on one's energy field or life force from a particular energy therapy; the fact that these interactions are in person simply explains, in part, why it is difficult to isolate the healing component in many energy therapies.

Energy Healing and Your Doctor

Some medical providers may be supportive of your decision to add energy therapies to your toolbox. In fact, many energy-healing studies have been conducted by physicians and nurses. Other medical providers may be unfamiliar with energy therapies, however. They may also assume that their effect is the result of a placebo response, and therefore not a "real" effect.

QUESTION

What is a placebo?
A placebo is an inactive "treatment," often used in research as a way of seeing whether a medication will work better than a "sugar pill" or "sham" treatment. Many people show genuine improvement when given the placebo, however, making the placebo effect a real one.

Finally, although many studies have found energy therapies to have a noticeable effect, many in the medical community have noted, not unfairly, that a number of these trials have been small or not well designed. There is much more to learn about how energy therapies may work, for which people and conditions, and which therapies are the most helpful. Following you will read about several of the more commonly used energy therapies, and ultimately you will have to decide for yourself whether any feel right for you. The good news is that these treatments pose little to no risk, may in fact be therapeutic, and quite possibly can facilitate healing on levels beyond an energetic one.

Hands-On Energy Healing

A number of energy-healing practices involve the transmission or manipulation of energy via a practitioner's hands, whether directly on or a few inches above the body. Some of the more well-known ones include Reiki, Therapeutic Touch, and Healing Touch, but certainly there are many others that are beyond the scope of this book to cover.

Anecdotally, people receiving these therapies commonly report an increased sense of peace and well-being, decreased worry, feeling comforted, and many report feeling like they can sleep better after a treatment.

Many also report feeling increased comfort in areas of their bodies that have felt tight, tense, or uncomfortable. Some even report experiences of enhanced spiritual connection.

Hands-on energetic practices can be performed on people of any age, as well as on animals, for the purposes of facilitating healing and increasing comfort. These therapies can be used to maintain feelings of well-being for those who are healthy, provide supportive care when someone is ill, and even provide comfort at the end of life. For this reason, many hospice facilities around the country offer some form of energy healing or are at least open to families bringing in their own energy healers to help loved ones through the dying process.

FACT

If you have never had an energy-healing session, and want to learn more before considering a treatment, you can view a demonstration video about Healing Touch (*https://www.youtube.com/watch?v=2mAqTTAyXcQ*). This video also summarizes the research and has commentary from health professionals.

Reiki

According to The International Center for Reiki Training, the name Reiki is made up of two Japanese words: "Rei," referring to a "higher power," and "Ki," which refers to "life force energy." Reiki is a technique for promoting healing via balancing life force energy, usually via laying hands on specific areas of one's own or another's body. Reiki can also be performed at a distance from the intended recipient. The premise of Reiki as a healing method is that when life force energy is low or out of balance, you may feel ill or more stressed.

Conversely, when this energy is balanced, your overall well-being will be enhanced and your physical and emotional health should be better. Reiki was brought from Japan to the Western world in the late 1930s, and recently has been increasingly integrated into healthcare and hospice settings.

Reiki sessions usually last thirty to forty-five minutes, but can be longer or shorter in duration. Typically, the practitioner will ask you some questions about your current state of health and what you hope to have addressed during the session. Then you will lie down on a massage table and the healer will work on you with her hands on or slightly above your body. You will remain fully clothed and may very well doze off during a treatment. If the practitioner is also trained in another CAM therapy, such as massage or reflexology, she may channel healing energy at the same time as she is providing the other service.

FACT

Doing regular self-healing is considered essential for Reiki practitioners, and many people pursue Reiki training solely to learn this practice. You can view a self-healing demonstration video by visiting *www.youtube.com/watch?v=W5HeyMeC468*.

Who Can Provide Reiki?

Reiki can be taught to people of all ages, regardless of spiritual tradition. Many people complete the first level of Reiki training simply to learn how to do self-Reiki, or self-healing, as that is the goal of beginning Reiki. Level I training involves taking in-person classes with a teacher referred to as a Reiki master, and in many cases can be achieved within a weekend or even less time. The next level of training, Reiki II, teaches you how to work on others both in person and at a distance. The highest level of training is that of Reiki master, and requires both in-person training and apprenticeship to another master teacher for an extended period of time. Each level of training is characterized in part by learning about and working with specific Reiki symbols. Upon completion of each level of training, the Reiki practitioner receives a certificate denoting this achievement.

Even with this general route to Reiki certification, however, there is some variation with regard to how each Reiki master trains students. There is also variability regarding the cost for trainings and the subsequent apprenticeship to a Reiki master. Furthermore, there are different schools of Reiki, so the teaching may vary with regard to hand placements and their order, and even the symbols used. The Reiki Alliance (*www.reikialliance.com/en*) is an organization of Reiki Masters who adhere to the Usui system of Reiki, which is considered to be closest to the way Reiki was originally taught.

Is Reiki a hands-on or distant-healing approach?
Reiki can actually be performed either in person or at a distance. Furthermore, Reiki can be performed either with the hands a few inches above the body or directly on it.

How to Find a Reiki Practitioner

In an effort to standardize Reiki training, both to achieve consistency of practice and make it easier to study scientifically, Reiki Master William Lee Rand established The International Center for Reiki Training and created an advisory board of scientists and nurses to facilitate further research into this therapy. Mr. Rand's system deviates to some degree from the original Usui system, as do the other variants. For more information, visit *www.reikimembership.com*. There are many other systems of Reiki that have evolved in the century since Reiki was brought to the West. A discussion of the various schools is beyond the scope of this book, however.

Because there is no national credentialing organization to oversee the quality of all Reiki training, as with a large number of CAM specialties, you will benefit from asking others you trust about Reiki practitioners they'd recommend. As a growing number of health professionals, such as nurses and licensed massage therapists, also are trained in some form of energy work, you may find practitioners who can combine Reiki or other energy-healing treatments with another health-related service.

ESSENTIAL

The Center for Reiki Research provides information about relevant research, and also lists a number of hospitals that offer Reiki. Additionally, the site links to other information about the practice. Membership is free. Visit *www.centerforreikiresearch.org*.

Phoebe Reclaiming Herself

Phoebe's diabetic peripheral neuropathy led to numbness, pins and needles, and sharp pains in both feet. She grieved the loss of a comfortable body and being able to walk easily. A neighbor recommended she try energy healing, and told her about Myra, a friend who was also a Reiki practitioner.

"I'm not sure I believe in that stuff," Phoebe said, "but I figure, what have I got to lose at this point? I'll try anything if it might help."

When Myra arrived to work on her, Phoebe expressed her doubts that Reiki could help, but said she was willing to keep an open mind. Halfway into the one-hour session, Phoebe was more comfortable and nearly asleep when Myra said, "Phoebe, the energy feels blocked as I move down your legs to your feet. Does that make sense?"

This observation surprised Phoebe, and she was further surprised when Myra continued, "The impression I get is that you have a lot of grief and resentment about your diabetes. I think you feel really overwhelmed by guilt as well."

By this point, Phoebe was tearful and simply nodded. Myra then said, "I think a lot of your distress and guilt and resentment have been directed at your feet, as if they have failed you. This cuts off energy flow to your feet. You need to forgive yourself for whatever decisions you made about how you took care of yourself before, and remember that however your feet are now, they are still a part of you. So you need to keep the energy flowing to them. Just breathe and imagine sending love and acceptance to all parts of you—feet included."

After the session finished, Phoebe slept better than she had in some time. Myra's words stayed with her, and Phoebe tried to imagine sending love to all parts of her. After a few more sessions with Myra, Phoebe decided to take a Level 1 Reiki training so she could balance her own energy. She began taking better care of herself in general, and felt more accepting of and at peace with the body she had. Her pain severity decreased somewhat and her coping improved. Phoebe had reclaimed herself.

Therapeutic Touch

Therapeutic Touch, or "TT," was developed in the 1970s by Dolores Krieger, a professor of nursing, and Dora Kunz, an energy healer. Dr. Krieger worked to standardize TT to make it easier to study. TT was originally designed as a helping practice and primarily taught in nursing education programs; however, practitioners also came from a variety of healthcare disciplines such as occupational and physical therapy, medicine, and nursing.

The founders considered healing work to be a universal human potential, and thus the training was opened to include non-healthcare professionals. As with Reiki, TT pairs well with other CAM therapies. After an initial consultation, the TT practitioner will assess the state of your energy field and then work to clear and rebalance it.

According to the Therapeutic Touch International Association, TT states that human beings are energy in the form of a field, and that the human energy field extends beyond the boundaries of the human body. Therapeutic Touch practitioners attune themselves to that energy using the hands as sensors, and then rebalance the energy accordingly. Sessions tend to average about twenty minutes in length, but can be longer or shorter depending on the needs of the individual.

Not only can biofield energy healing be performed on people of all ages, but it can also be done for animals, from family pets, to shelter animals, to horses and zoo animals. Practitioners often report that animals quickly become very relaxed and peaceful when having an energy healing session.

Who Can Provide Therapeutic Touch?

Becoming a TT practitioner requires completing basic and intermediate levels of training. If a practitioner wants to achieve the next level of training and teach, she must do additional training and apprentice with a teacher. One can become a practitioner without necessarily going on to teach, however.

TT certification is more formalized and centralized than the training for Reiki is, and requires applying for credentialing to the Therapeutic Touch International Association. Renewals are for a four-year period only. Teachers must complete advanced training and also engage in approved continuing education in the form of classes, conferences, and workshops on a yearly basis. Therapeutic Touch International Associates (TTIA) education programs are approved through the American Holistic Nurses Association or other American Association of Critical-Care Nurses (AACN) providers, such as state nursing associations. For more information on this process, visit *http://therapeutic-touch.org/credentialing.*

How to Find a TT Practitioner

The Therapeutic Touch International Association maintains a list of certified teachers throughout the US. Visit *http://therapeutic-touch.org/about-us/qualified-teachers/* to find a teacher near you, or *http://therapeutic-touch.org/about-us/qualified-practitioner/* to find a TT practitioner in your area.

Healing Touch

Janet Mentgen, who sought to expand the connections between nurses and their patients, founded Healing Touch. She saw the positive effect of touch while serving as a nurse in the U.S. Navy in emergency room settings, and then in home healthcare. Mentgen developed a Healing Touch certificate program that has since been endorsed by the American Holistic Nurses Association, the Canadian Holistic Nurses Association, and other health-related organizations. Healing Touch training has become available internationally.

Like TT and Reiki, Healing Touch practitioners use their hands to sense, clear, energize, and balance the energy field in an effort to improve physical, emotional, mental, and spiritual health. Clients lie fully clothed on a massage table while the practitioner first speaks with the client to assess his concerns and current health status, before commencing the energy work. Hands can be placed a few inches above or directly on the client's body during a treatment.

To become a practitioner, students of Healing Touch must complete five levels of coursework and receive a certificate of completion, as well as apprentice with a mentor for a minimum of a year. Students must then submit an application and achieve a passing score on a proficiency exam. The Healing Touch Program credentials students who have met these requirements as certified. This credential must be renewed every five years. Practitioners may then decide whether to become an instructor, which requires additional training and a formal application process. The curriculum and requirements are tailored to health professionals, but Healing Touch training is open to those outside the health professions provided they document either college-level course work in relevant areas, or equivalent other training.

More information is available about this healing modality on the Healing Touch Program website, *www.healingtouchprogram.com*, including how to locate a certified practitioner or instructor (*www.htpractitioner.com*).

What the Science Says about Energy Therapies

The official statement by NCCIH says that there is too little data, and problems with the design of many existing studies, to say for certain whether Reiki is an effective therapy for any medical condition. In terms of scientific support for their use, a 2010 review of biofield studies published in the *International Journal of Behavioral Medicine* examined the research on Reiki, Therapeutic Touch, and Healing Touch. The authors concluded that biofield therapies showed strong evidence for reducing pain intensity in those with chronic pain, and moderate evidence for reducing pain intensity in hospitalized and cancer populations. The results were somewhat mixed with regard to the impact on anxiety and depression in those with chronic pain. In some studies, biofield therapies seemed to have a positive impact, and in others, the impact was not significant. In general, the authors concluded that biofield therapies can help decrease pain intensity, increase quality of life related to physical functioning, and may help you feel better overall. This review can be accessed via *www.ncbi.nlm.nih.gov/pmc/articles/PMC2816237*.

A 2014 review of Reiki alone published in the journal *Pain Management Nursing* focused on results from seven high-quality studies that examined the impact of receiving Reiki for anxiety or pain. The authors concluded that Reiki may be effective for reducing pain and anxiety, but, again, that more, high-quality research was needed.

Some Healing Touch studies have found this approach associated with pain reduction, reduced fatigue, decreased stress, and improved mood, improvements in blood pressure, heart rate, relaxation, and well-being. And a recent study found benefits for reducing pain and improving physical function in knee osteoarthritis, as well as decreased depression.

The results from energy-healing research are mixed, with some studies showing measurable benefits and some not. Most of these studies are small, and thus it's difficult to generalize their findings to pain patients. That said, energy healing appears to be safe and should not be cost prohibitive for the average person, particularly if the method used is for self-healing.

Tips on Choosing an Energy Healer

After you have asked friends and healthcare providers for recommendations, or done Internet searches for energy healers in your area, choosing the practitioner that is right for you should come down to the following:

- **Do you feel comfortable with this person?** Trust your feelings when meeting any provider. Does this person seem compassionate, attentive, and committed to helping you heal? Do you have a good rapport with this person? The latter can be hard to define, but you know when you feel safe and understood by another. If for some reason the connection just does not feel right, it's unlikely you will be able to relax enough to fully enjoy and benefit from the sessions.
- **Assess the person's experience with healing.** It's perfectly acceptable to ask, "How long have you been doing energy work?" "What led you to this field?" "Are you trained in any other healing modalities?"
- **Assess affordability.** Rates for individual energy-healing sessions can vary by geographic location, modality, and the practitioner's level of experience. That said, fees for an energy-healing session should neither be exorbitant nor beyond what you can afford. If finances are a concern for you, ask whether a sliding scale is possible. If not, inquire about healing circles that are open to the public, many of which are free or low cost.

An Internet search of practitioners in your area can give you an idea of what the average rate is for a particular therapy. For the most part, energy-healing sessions, particularly by a provider who is not also licensed in a healthcare discipline such as nursing or who is not providing a dual service (e.g., energy healing plus massage, physical therapy, or acupuncture) should not exceed the fee for any of your medical providers (and should probably be more affordable)— no matter how long the practitioner has worked in her discipline.

Exercises to Sense the Energy Field

Most energy-healing systems are based on the premise that anyone can learn to do energy healing, and thus can learn to feel or balance his *own* energy. The following are a few simple exercises to help you become familiar with sensing energy. You might find you get the best results initially by trying them in order. Although everyone perceives energy a bit differently, you may notice feeling the energy field as a slight resistance against the hand you use to sense it. You might also notice a change in temperature, or a pleasant, lightly prickly or mildly electric sensation, either in the hand you use for sensing or the part being sensed, or both. At first, the sensations may be extremely subtle or difficult to detect. You may wish to prepare with a few minutes of mindfulness or gentle breathing to help you clear your mind and get comfortable. Try to simply remain open-minded, relaxed, and enjoy the experience. Write down your observations.

- *Sensing the "Qi Ball"*—First, briskly rub your palms together for a few moments, and then relax your hands and arms. With the rest of your body comfortably relaxed, whether standing or seated, now hold your hands out in front of you, elbows at your sides, palms open, a few inches apart and facing each other, as if you were holding a small ball between them. Simply notice what you observe, whether something significant, subtle, or nothing at all. Imagine you are inhaling and exhaling through your hands with each breath. While still maintaining space between your hands, bring your palms to within about an inch of each other. Slide your hands slowly forward and back . . . then bring them slightly farther apart, then back again, and apart once more, as if you had a piece of taffy between them that you were gently stretching and contracting. If you sense the energy field, perhaps as warmth or tingling or static electricity, notice how far apart you can move your palms before the feeling diminishes. Some people find that they wind up with a very sizable qi ball. Whatever you notice is perfectly fine.
- *Sensing Your Lung Meridian*—In Traditional Chinese Medicine, the lung meridian is fairly easy to sense with the hands. This meridian runs from just inside your shoulder (near where your chest and shoulder meet) down the inside of your arm and to the tip of your thumb. Begin by deciding which lung meridian you want to sense, and hold that arm out in front of you in a relaxed manner, with the thumb-side of your hand closest to the ceiling (as if you were about to shake someone's hand, but with your arm and hand relaxed). Without making contact, take your other hand and simply move it slowly down from your shoulder, over your upper arm

and then the inside of your elbow, all the way down to the tip of your thumb, again, just noticing what you observe. Move your hand slowly back up towards your shoulder, and notice if the sensation in either the sensing hand or the arm being sensed changes as you bring the two closer or farther apart. Does the sensation change when your hand is over your hand and thumb versus over your arm or shoulder?

- *Sensing Another's Lung Meridian*—Once you've become familiar with sensing your own energy field, try sensing the field of another person (with their permission, of course!). Remaining at least an inch or two away from the other person's meridian, again move your hand up to the shoulder and then back down over the thumb. Note how this person's energy field feels compared to sensing your own. If you find yourself trying too hard to feel the energy field, and have little success at first, there is no need to worry. You can always take a break and return your awareness to your breath to clear your mind. Remember, just like using your "normal senses," it tends to work better if you "let" rather than "try." (You don't "try" to smell a cake baking or see the color of a flower, right?) You can also allow part of your awareness to stay with your breathing while the other half of your attention is engaged in these exercises. Above all, see these practices as opportunities to relax, try something new, and enjoy without having to "succeed" at them.

Homeopathy

Chances are, you have come across homeopathic remedies at your local health food store, natural foods market, and even at chain drugstores. Homeopathic cold and flu remedies, sleep aids, and preparations for pain relief are among the most common remedies you'll notice, although homeopathic remedies seem to exist for nearly any ailment one could imagine.

Homeopathy is the name given to an alternative medical system that was developed in Germany about 200 years ago. A primary premise of homeopathy is that "like cures like," or that an illness or symptom can be cured by a tiny dose of something that would normally produce those symptoms. The second, related premise is that the smaller the dose of that substance, the more potent the treatment is.

Homeopathic preparations come in liquid, cream, gel, or tablet forms, and an alternative health provider will typically individualize the treatment to the person. Popular homeopathic remedies for pain include arnica, which is also thought to reduce bruising, and a preparation called Traumeel. Traumeel was developed by a German physician in the 1930s, and contains a number of herbal and other ingredients. Some of these ingredients you may recognize, such as arnica, chamomile, witch hazel, St. John's wort, and calendula. It also contains belladonna, which in larger quantities is deadly, but when extremely dilute is thought to contribute to pain relief. Traumeel is purported to have anti-inflammatory, as well as pain-relieving properties, and to reduce swelling.

FACT

According to the NCCIH and data from the 2012 National Health Interview Survey, homeopathic remedies are among the most popular CAM therapies used in the US. In fact, adults spent about $2.9 billion on homeopathic remedies and $170 million on visits to homeopathic providers.

What the Science Says

Homeopathy remains one of the more controversial CAM therapies, as the basic assumptions of this approach are counter to generally accepted scientific principles. The NCCIH has concluded, based on the available research, that the evidence suggests that homeopathy is not an effective therapy in general. Despite this position, at this writing, a multicenter trial is underway comparing dexamethasone (a steroid) and Traumeel injections for the treatment of rotator cuff pain.

A 2013 study comparing Traumeel ointment, Traumeel gel, and diclofenac gel (an NSAID pain reliever) for pain due to severe ankle sprain found that the Traumeel products reduced pain and improved mobility as well as the drug did. Other studies of patients with musculoskeletal injuries have found an association between Traumeel and reduced pain, improved mobility, and reduced swelling as compared to a placebo (sham) treatment. Traumeel also seems to be well tolerated and the adverse responses are reportedly rare and mild (e.g., transient skin reactions such as redness and itching).

ALERT

Some homeopathic preparations are recommended as substitutes for vaccination; however, to date, there is not scientific evidence supporting this claim. If you have questions about immunization, visit *www.vaccines.gov* for more information.

There is some, but less, evidence suggesting that arnica preparations help reduce pain. One study found that arnica gel was as effective as ibuprofen in improving pain and hand function in patients with osteoarthritis of the hand. Another small study found that arnica was more effective than placebo at reducing pain after carpal tunnel surgery. At least one in-vitro study (involving samples of cells) found that arnica seemed to have anti-inflammatory effects. Although the results of a few studies are intriguing, at present the majority of scientific data do not show significant benefits associated with using arnica.

Although, traditionally, homeopathic remedies are so diluted that few or even no molecules of the original substances remain and therefore there should be no possibility of harm, some remedies labeled homeopathic may contain high enough amounts of certain substances to be harmful. Also, liquid homeopathic preparations may contain alcohol, and as such may interact with some of the other medications you are prescribed.

Overall, more, higher-quality studies would need to be performed to definitively recommend most homeopathic remedies for pain or other ailments. Traumeel seems to have a good safety profile and enough evidence of benefit to make it low risk and possibly of benefit. That said, avoid alcohol-based preparations if you are currently taking medications that may interact negatively with alcohol.

If you choose to use homeopathic remedies, seek the counsel of a physician who is trained and experienced in using them and is familiar with which brands are reputable and safe. Those that are appropriately diluted are most probably safe to use, effective or not. Naturopathic doctors, or NDs, are more likely to be familiar with homeopathy than conventional medical doctors, and therefore can make a personalized recommendation based on your health status and goals for treatment. NDs can work as licensed physicians in some states. The American Association of Naturopathic Physicians maintains a list of states where NDs can be licensed. The site also maintains information on a variety of natural remedies, including homeopathy.

CHAPTER 13

Cognitive-Behavioral Therapy

Cognitive-behavioral therapy, or CBT, is a psychotherapy approach that takes into account the relationship between your thoughts, feelings, and behaviors. It provides a framework for changing patterns, learning new ways of coping, and has been shown to help with managing pain and the mood symptoms and stress so often associated with a painful condition. CBT is considered a first-line psychosocial treatment for chronic pain for both adults and children. Therefore, it is technically a "conventional" treatment, even though it is also a nonmedical and a mind-body one.

Why CBT?

CBT is considered an "empirically validated" treatment, meaning that CBT's usefulness for helping manage a variety of conditions has been demonstrated in a number of studies. For example, in addition to helping with chronic pain, CBT is considered effective for treating posttraumatic stress, panic, obsessive-compulsive disorder, eating disorders, bipolar disorder, schizophrenia, generalized anxiety, borderline personality, and depression.

Unlike some other forms of therapy, CBT is typically time-limited, in that treatment takes place over a specific number of sessions, rather than being open-ended in length. That said, treatment can, in many cases, continue beyond the short term if needed. For example, you may begin seeing a CBT therapist to learn how to manage pain, and as you achieve your goals you might decide to set new goals, such as decreasing anxiety related to public speaking, developing more effective communication skills, or decreasing fear related to flying.

CBT techniques and principles can also be incorporated into integrative psychotherapy frameworks, and thus the overall treatment may be less structured and more open-ended with regard to the time frame. An integrative psychotherapy approach draws on the strengths of different psychotherapy models and possibly other healing traditions so that the work is further tailored to the individual's needs and the therapist's preferred way of working.

Thoughts, Feelings, and Behaviors, Oh My!

A simple but important principle related to CBT says that your thoughts, feelings, and behaviors (or choices) are all linked. Specifically, your thoughts tend to affect both your feelings and the subsequent decisions you make. Similarly, your feelings affect the type or quality of the thoughts you have, and what you ultimately decide to do in an effort to feel better.

For example, if you have a presentation coming up at work and you are feeling anxious about it (the emotion), you might think, "What if they think my presentation is awful?" or "What if someone asks me a question I can't answer?" These types of thoughts will probably increase your anxiety.

Depending on the coping skills or tool you typically use, you might do something like try to reframe the thoughts ("Actually, I know my material well. It's normal to be nervous before giving a talk, but that doesn't mean it won't go well. I have prepared and will do just fine."). Reframing, even though it is an internal process, is also a type of behavior or action that can be very helpful.

If your anxiety gets the better of you, or if you are used to using avoidance as a coping tool, you may decide to cancel your presentation instead. Avoidance often works in the short term because once the anxiety-provoking event is canceled, your anxiety will almost certainly decrease. Ultimately, however, avoiding anxiety-provoking situations will actually increase your anxiety when you finally must do something that you've gotten out of doing previously.

Avoiding things prevents you from getting used to (or becoming desensitized to) them, and also deprives you of an opportunity for success. Each time you are successful, you will poke holes in the argument that you cannot do something or can't do it well enough. So, the thought "I can't do this" can lead to feelings of anxiety, but what you choose to do can be either adaptive (e.g., reframing, or choosing a different strategy) or unhelpful (e.g., running away from the situation).

Another adaptive option for dealing with stress might be to go for a walk, engage in relaxation exercises, or call a friend. Each of these things is likely to help you feel better by becoming more relaxed and less worried. As you feel less worried and more relaxed from your walk, or spending time with your friends, your thoughts will probably also become less catastrophic and more realistic. But, as you can see, your thoughts and feelings will affect each other and what you decide to do at any given time.

Behavioral Activation: A Tool for Feeling Better

"Behavioral activation" is a term that simply means engaging in activities that help you feel better. Your CBT therapist may mention this to you or you may decide to include this in your pain- and mood-management plan. Behavioral activation has been shown to improve mood, and is another way you can take the reins back from pain. The steps for doing this are very simple.

1. Think of the health-supportive activities, choices, and behaviors that tend to help you feel relaxed, happy, or fulfilled.
2. If it seems difficult to come up with a list at first, over the course of the next week keep a pain and mood diary to track how your symptoms and emotions change depending on what you are doing.

3. After reviewing your diary, jot down a list of the activities that helped you feel more relaxed, less stressed, happier, or helped move your pain into the background. Common examples include spending time with loved ones, going for a walk, engaging in a creative activity (e.g., painting, drawing, singing, dance), volunteering to help others, doing yoga stretches, meditating, using aromatherapy, etc.

4. Schedule the pleasant activities into your week, just as you would any other important event or obligation. This will ensure you make time for them and make it more likely that you will follow through with them.

5. Do the activities! Do them even if a part of you resists doing them or questions if they will really be helpful, and do them even if you are tired or discouraged. Do not wait until your pain "goes away" or goes down below a level it normally reaches (if you wait for this time to come, you may find yourself never doing the activities you schedule, and ultimately feeling worse). *If you have scheduled it, do it.*

6. Keep a journal of how you felt right before, during, right after, and a few hours after the activity. Use a numerical system to rate your pain, mood, and fatigue. The zero-to-ten system (where zero is "no symptom" and ten is "the worst symptom severity possible") is useful for most people, but if you prefer, you can simply note "mild," "moderate," or "severe."

7. At the end of the week, note which activities seem to be most effective. Schedule these into the following week, and keep those very important "appointments!"

CBT can also help you shed light on some of the "core beliefs" and "automatic thoughts" that have been shaping how you view yourself and the world, and can help you set and achieve goals in a stepwise manner. Goals can be related to managing your emotions, such as decreasing depressive symptoms; changing the way you do things, such as eating a healthier diet; or shifting your perspective, such as changing a tendency to catastrophize.

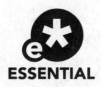

ESSENTIAL

Reframing is a simple but powerful CBT technique that helps you step back from stressful thoughts, put them in perspective, and view them in a more realistic and positive light. Reframing can help you decrease stress and increase confidence. With practice, reframing will become easier and easier.

What CBT Is

If you have been in therapy before, you may have a specific idea of what sessions will be like; however, CBT is different from traditional talk therapy (e.g., psychodynamic psychotherapy) in a number of ways. Here are some characteristics of CBT treatments:

- *CBT is collaborative.* Your therapist will partner with you to help you determine what you want to change, and come up with a plan to make this happen.
- *CBT is structured.* You and your therapist will discuss your broad goals for treatment (e.g., becoming more active), come up with more specific goals (running five miles), the steps you will take to achieve your goals (begin by walking five days a week for ten minutes per day), and identify what things currently make it easier or more difficult to do this (scheduling exercise before other family members wake up).
- *CBT is typically time-limited.* Your treatment may take place over a predetermined number of sessions, such as over the course of twelve or sixteen weeks. If needed, you may continue working with your therapist on the original goal, or perhaps set new ones.
- *Your therapist will be active.* She will ask and respond to questions, and provide different tools and exercises geared toward helping you make the changes you desire. Examples include in-session role-playing to help you rehearse doing a new behavior or communicating effectively, helping you identify beliefs that may be holding you back, leading you in guided imagery exercises, or teaching you relaxation techniques.
- *You will need to be active.* CBT typically involves some homework outside the sessions to help you learn more about pain triggers and alleviators, understand barriers and facilitators to engaging in healthy behaviors, and also practice stress-reduction techniques. Homework will reinforce what you learn in sessions and further help you chart your progress and accomplish your goals. For CBT to work for you, you will need to be willing to do some work.
- *CBT is geared to the present.* Although you and your therapist will work together to understand the origins of limiting beliefs, behaviors, and patterns, the major focus will be on helping you use this information to feel better and make positive changes in the present.

- *CBT pairs well with many other approaches.* Mindfulness, guided imagery, hypnosis, relaxation training, and biofeedback can be easily incorporated into a CBT session. Furthermore, aromatherapy can be paired with a number of CBT techniques to further enhance the experience of relaxation.

ESSENTIAL

In the short term, avoidance "works," because it tends to make anxiety decrease. But in the long term, avoiding things that may provoke anxiety but that you really need to do actually makes it harder to do them in the future. Your mind and body will "expect" you to stop doing things that stress you out.

Dylan's "Prison"

Dylan was a competitive tennis player and the captain of his high school tennis team. Dylan experienced stabbing, hot, neuropathic pain in his right shoulder that resulted in $10/10$, or "the worst imaginable" pain spikes, and $8/10$ average pain. After an intensive course of physical therapy and medication, Dylan's average pain decreased to $2/10$, spiking to $6/10$ once or twice per week for a few minutes each time, usually after he'd been working on the computer for too long.

A pain diary helped Dylan realize that he actually had many times when his pain seemed barely noticeable or even absent—a very good result given his condition. Dylan struggled with constant sadness, anger, and resentment that he had *any* pain, however, and even minimal pain generated significant catastrophizing. "I feel like I'm a prisoner in my own body! I watch other people playing tennis like I used to, and I just feel trapped in here." Dylan's greatest source of distress was that he was no longer able to compete at the level he could prior to his accident.

"I can't believe this is still going on!" At times, Dylan was despondent. "I don't even see the point in living if I can't compete. That's just who I am. This is *the worst thing that could possibly happen*! No one understands." Dylan's catastrophizing could also be referred to as his *automatic thoughts* about his situation.

Dylan's distress persisted despite the fact that he was able to return to playing tennis, albeit at a less competitive level. In therapy, Dylan revealed that he knew that although he had been a great high school tennis player, even at his best he was not playing at the level of a professional athlete. Therefore, after college, his tennis would have become solely recreational, even if he had never been injured and was not in pain. Dylan's rational mind knew that his worth was not determined by his tennis prowess, but another part of him believed that without being a tennis "great," his worth as a person was diminished.

In CBT sessions, Dylan became aware that he held a core belief that unless he was "the best," he would be "nothing." Dylan was able to link this belief to the fact that although his parents loved him, he was typically only praised for stellar athletic achievements, and tennis in particular, rather than simply for putting forth effort, or for any inherent quality. "I guess I never thought I could be worth something unless I was really *great*—you know, competitive, and actually winning at something."

Doing a hierarchy of fears during the first sessions, with zero indicating no fear and 100 representing the most fearful, awful situation he could imagine, Dylan had indicated that never again playing tennis competitively in high school or when at college would rate as "100—absolutely! I can't even think of anything worse than that." When he revisited this exercise several weeks later, however, Dylan was able to reframe this situation. "Actually, I really, really *want* to play competitively again. And I'm so angry and sad that I'm not where I was before, and maybe I won't ever be. But there are other things I can imagine that would be worse than not competing. Losing a family member, not being able to do all of the things I can still do physically, losing my best friend—those things would actually be worse." Dylan learned to identify cognitive distortions like catastrophizing and challenge them.

In addition, Dylan found that several techniques helped him cope with his situation and do things to make life better in the present. Mindfulness helped him notice thoughts and feelings without attaching to them or automatically assuming they were "true;" diaphragmatic breathing helped him calm down when he noticed his anxiety or fear rising; and behavioral activation, or engaging in pleasurable activities, helped him improve mood symptoms. In essence, he had used his mind to set himself free.

CBT for Pain Management

By now, you know quite a bit about why mind-body approaches can help your brain turn down the volume on pain. The research on CBT for pain has found that CBT can help decrease pain severity, improve coping, help you understand what things trigger or alleviate pain, reduce disability from pain, decrease catastrophizing, increase engagement in positive health behaviors, improve mood and quality of life, and decrease headache frequency, to name some of the benefits. CBT can also help you reach other goals that are important for managing pain and helping you to feel better, including general stress management, losing weight or improving your eating habits, getting better sleep, and the like.

The Hierarchy of Fears

As you saw in the example with Dylan, your fears about pain, your body, or your functioning can become catastrophic. This level of fear and catastrophizing has been shown to make your pain worse, not better, however, and also worsens mood. It's important to challenge the ideas you have about what would be "intolerable!" or "the most terrible thing ever!" Challenging these ideas does not mean that you have to think difficult things are "hunky-dory" or totally fine. But it is essential to put them into perspective so you can make the best of the life and body you have at any given time, as you continue to work toward making positive change.

Hierarchy of Fears

Note the thing that seems like something you absolutely could not tolerate or survive related to your pain or health. Draw a vertical line, with 0 at the left and 100 at the right. The zero represents no fear, while the 100 represents your worst fear imaginable. Make a vertical mark in the line representing where this falls on the line. Don't overthink it, just put the mark where it feels like it belongs for now.

Next, either right after doing this, or after taking a little time to reflect further, think of other things that you feel would be extremely difficult to tolerate. Make a second line and mark that line to represent these things or events. When you are done, see where the item from the first hierarchy would fit in among those items in the second. Is the original fear in the same place, or has its position changed? Reflect on what this means for you.

The Pain Diary

You've already learned about using a pain diary to chart when you have pain, what internal or external factors seem to trigger it, the thoughts and emotions associated with the triggers, as well as what action you took to change your pain and what the result was. Keeping a pain diary is important, at least in the beginning of your pain management journey, for a number of reasons.

First, becoming aware of what typically triggers your pain can help you make more informed choices. As an example, if you find that consuming alcohol usually triggers a migraine, next time you go out, you will be able to consciously choose whether to have that glass of wine—and the migraine— or whether you will want to forgo what one part of you may desire because the larger part of you feels it may not be worth the cost (a migraine). Understanding your pain triggers can put you in the driver's seat and alleviate some of the helplessness often associated with chronic pain.

Relatedly, keeping track of the actions you take to alleviate your pain, and then rating the pain severity afterward, can shed light on whether a treatment is working, and if so, how well. Remember, a change of two points on a ten-point scale, or 20 percent, is considered a clinically meaningful result. You can then weigh the pros and cons of whether the benefits of that result are worth the costs, and vice versa. For example, if taking an opioid pain medicine results in a three-point decrease in your back pain, you may decide it is helpful to continue with that medication. If taking it also results in significant constipation or feeling "out of it," you may decide that the degree of relief you experience is not worth the "cost" of the medication's side effects, and then discuss alternatives with your doctor.

CBT Terms

The following italicized words are common terms used in CBT. Knowing what they mean and how they relate to your treatment will help you better understand your healing process:

- *Core beliefs* are thoughts a person has that determine how he views himself and the world around him. Core beliefs are like lenses that every thought, feeling, and experience are viewed through. There are positive core beliefs (e.g., "I know I have inherent worth") that will not likely be ones you spend much time exploring, and which you will not want to change. Core beliefs that cause frequent distress, or get in the way of normal, healthy functioning, whether professionally, academically, socially, emotionally, or otherwise (e.g., "I am stupid" or "I am only lovable when I achieve things") are important to recognize and challenge. A way to do this is to examine the evidence for and against them. For example, a student may believe he is basically stupid, but evidence to the contrary may be that he has a B average, does well on exams when he studies, knows a great deal about his favorite sport (i.e., evidence he can learn), etc.

- *Automatic thoughts* are thoughts one has reflexively in response to certain situations. Core beliefs shape the automatic thoughts you will have—even if you are not yet consciously aware of what your core beliefs are. For example, the student who has a core belief that he is stupid will probably think, "Oh, I only did well on that test because it was easy; everybody probably did well." People tend to assume that their automatic thoughts represent "truth," yet these may be driven by erroneous core beliefs.

- *Feelings*, or your emotions, such as sadness, anger, grief, anxiety, etc., both influence the types of thoughts you have, and are influenced by your thoughts. For example, when you are depressed, everything in your world may seem pointless to you. And when you think you are being treated unfairly, you will likely feel angry.

- *Behaviors* represent the things you *do*, whether they are active (such as smoking when you are stressed versus going for a walk) or passive (avoiding situations that make you anxious). Your thoughts and feelings influence the behaviors you choose to do (or not do). In addition, many behaviors will help you change the way you think and feel. The consensus is that it is actually easier to start with changing a behavior (i.e., doing something different) than it is to try to change a thought. And it's easier to directly change a thought than it is to change a feeling. Behavioral activation is one example of a tool that can help you change your thoughts and emotions, and feel better in general, by choosing to engage in a specific behavior.

Pros and Cons

After keeping a pain diary for a week or so, you may want to re-examine whether to continue an existing strategy or adopt a new one based on how your pain responds to what you normally do and the other factors associated with this tool.

Think of a behavior or tool you have used or are considering using to help manage pain, sadness, anxiety, fear, etc., that a part of you wonders whether you should use, or has had trouble sticking with. This might be something most people would say you should discontinue, like smoking; alternatively, it might be something that generally would be considered a healthy tool, but may also be one you are resistant to using for any number of reasons, such as increasing your exercise or engaging in physical therapy.

In the spaces that follow, write down the pros and cons in both the short- and long-term. Seeing these in "black and white" can help you commit firmly to a decision to begin, retain, change, or stop a behavior altogether:

BEHAVIOR OR TREATMENT IN QUESTION: [EX: SMOKING] _____

Pros (Short-Term) for Continuing	Cons (Short-Term) for Continuing
Ex: Something to do when I'm nervous	Partner hates smell; Cost per pack is high
_____	_____
_____	_____
_____	_____

Pros (Long-Term) for Continuing	Cons (Long-Term) for Continuing
Ex: Is a tool I'm used to and know it makes me feel less anxious in the moment; No need to invest time in learning another tool	Increased Cancer Risk; Annual expense is prohibitive
_____	_____
_____	_____
_____	_____

The Importance of Pacing

Pacing refers to having specific parameters with regard to rest and activity, so that you neither "under-do" nor "over-do" work or sleep. Chronic pain and the fatigue associated with it can lead to increased periods of rest and decreased activity and productivity. Because chronic pain spikes can interfere with your ability to do as much as you would otherwise, whether at work or at home, you may find yourself feeling guilty or anxious about the things that don't get done when you are feeling particularly ill.

As an example, if you experience a migraine, you may feel unable to attend a meeting at work, or choose to stay home altogether. Upon returning to the office, however, you may notice increased internal pressure to "catch up," and you may find yourself putting in extra hours upon recovery from the headache. After a series of late nights or working through weekends, you may find your migraines are back with a vengeance and your distress markedly increased. Similarly, if you have a Crohn's flare-up and your abdominal pain, diarrhea, or body aches interrupt your plans to clean and do laundry, you may become more and more distressed as the laundry piles up and chores go unfinished. After a few days of rest, you may find yourself trying to do ten loads of laundry instead of two or three, leaving you overwhelmed, exhausted, and once again in need of a rest period.

The cycle of inactivity/over-activity may be especially common and difficult for you to interrupt if your self-esteem is strongly linked to your performance at work, school, or with regard to how you keep your home. You may even find yourself in what psychologists refer to as a "double bind," a situation in which you feel there is no way you can win, or no good choice you can make.

In an earlier chapter, you saw how "Kenny" fell into this trap at his sales job, missing work due to migraines and then overcompensating by working extra hours, skipping lunch, and working weekends. He felt caught in a vicious cycle of debilitating headaches, missing work, increased stress, more overcompensation, and another cycle of severe headaches. Before long, Kenny realized he felt stressed and exhausted even when he wasn't having a migraine, and it took less and less work for him to require rest. Because his boss was unaware of what was going on, he assumed Kenny was simply a "feast or famine" type of employee—productive when he was "good," but overall unpredictable.

The Undone Do-It-Yourselfer

Bill was a father of three in his forties and a proud "do-it-yourselfer" who loved working on his house, biking, and camping on weekends. Bill developed Lyme disease after an extended trip of camping in the woods.

He later developed arthritis secondary to this illness, leaving him with joint pain and periods of significant fatigue. Not being able to do the things he loved as often as he used to left Bill feeling discouraged and depressed, as well as worried.

When Bill felt well, he tended to start larger-scale home improvement projects and go for extended bike rides. "I figure, I'd better get it in while I can. Because tomorrow I might feel pretty terrible, and then never get around to doing the things I love." Although Bill thought he was maximizing the times when he felt well, inevitably, a long bike ride or marathon home-improvement stint would trigger a spike in his arthritis and fatigue that left him unable to bike, work on his house, and sometimes do much of anything for a week or more. During these times, Bill's pain and frustration were much worse than normal. The idea of setting limits on his activities ahead of time made Bill feel like a "slouch." Eventually, however, Bill realized that by pacing, he could actually have *more* days of doing what he loved, even if he didn't do those activities as intensely or for as long as he did before he developed a pain syndrome.

Pacing requires you to determine what schedule of work and rest tends to keep your body—the one you have at present, rather than the one you had prior to your diagnosis—in better balance. It can help you have many more "good" and "productive" days overall, even if you do less each day than you used to.

Pacing, contrary to popular belief, is *not*:

- Working to the point of pain and then stopping
- Choosing to work to fatigue or the point of pain early in the day, and then dedicating the remainder of the day to resting
- Resting for the most part and doing as little as possible in general

It will take some time and observation to come up with the best plan for you. A good rule of thumb is to observe, in general, how much of a particular type of activity you can usually do, and for what amount of time, before you usually find yourself fatigued or in pain. If you typically notice that after cleaning your house for forty-five minutes you feel an increase in pain, fatigue, or both, you may decide to break tasks into thirty-minute blocks, alternating with periods of awake rest.

If you normally can walk or jog one mile before you begin to notice pain or tiredness, schedule regular activity but "quit while you are ahead," as they say, perhaps walking one-half or three-quarters of a mile so you can return home still feeling well enough to be present and awake for the remainder of the day, or with minimal rest. If you tend to get headaches when working on the computer, schedule stretch breaks every hour, or as often as you need to prevent pain spikes.

To effectively pace yourself:

- Keep a log or diary of rest, activity, and pain spikes. Look for the patterns so you can adjust your pacing accordingly.
- Let go of needing to be "Superman," or even "my old self." There is no such thing as being perfect, but there *is* such a thing as being effective. Successful people understand and work with their natural rhythms rather than fighting against them. This enables them to be effective.
- Redefine and embrace your successes. Decreasing the frequency, intensity, or duration of your pain flare-ups is an important type of success! Also, remember that people tend to be more productive in the long run by being consistent and moderate, rather than via a feast-or-famine, all-or-nothing approach.
- Allow the "rest" to be "restorative." Use the rest periods for gentle stretching, meditation, prayer, or other activities that are relaxing. Try to remain awake and relaxed, rather than sleeping during breaks, as this will help you maintain a normal sleep-wake cycle and feel less groggy during the day.
- As your health, fitness, or energy levels improve, you can experiment with gradually increasing your active time—in small, measurable increments, over a period of a few days or weeks. If you find you can maintain this new level, feel free to stay with it. If you find your pain cycling worsens, return to the pacing that keeps you involved in your life and feeling you can get things done without leaving you feeling depleted.

Relaxation Training

Relaxation training is a key component of CBT pain management. Relaxation practices can help you decrease stress and increase calm, thereby closing the pain gate. They can also help you decrease muscular tension and get back in touch with feelings of comfort in your body.

Hypnosis, guided imagery, biofeedback, and mindfulness can be incorporated into your CBT treatment as ways to induce the relaxation response and decrease pain. Other techniques include diaphragmatic breathing, "four-square" breathing, and progressive muscle relaxation.

Diaphragmatic Breathing

Diaphragmatic breathing, also referred to as belly breathing or abdominal breathing, involves training your body to take deeper, slower, more relaxing breaths. The diaphragm is a large muscle located between your chest and your abdomen. When you allow your belly to expand outward while inhaling, your diaphragm contracts, drawing more air into your lungs and thus providing you with more oxygen. This type of breathing also improves blood flow to your heart and facilitates the relaxation response. If you have ever watched babies sleep, you may have noticed that they naturally "do" abdominal breathing rather than breathing into their chests.

Typically, when you are stressed or anxious, or if you tend to have a hunched posture, you will expand your chest but not your belly when breathing. Luckily, belly breathing is easy to learn, and you will almost certainly feel more relaxed after doing even ten cycles of inhalation and exhalation this way. You can watch a brief animated illustration of diaphragmatic breathing here: *www.youtube.com/watch?v=1WMt_1jw47Q*. You can also follow these instructions:

Belly Breathing Exercise

If your muscles feel a bit tight, it may be helpful to do some gentle stretching beforehand. Then, sit comfortably, making sure your spine is fairly straight and your legs are uncrossed. Begin by noticing the natural rate and rhythm of your breath, however it is right in this moment. Place one hand on your lower abdomen and one hand on your chest. Just notice which hand tends to rise more—the one on your chest or the one on your belly.

Breathing in through your nose and out through your mouth, notice the difference in how it feels to breathe when your chest does the expanding, versus when you allow your belly to expand with the "in" breath and relax with the "out" breath. With your awareness still on your breathing, gently but deliberately breathe into your belly, visualizing this, if you like. Feel the easy rise of the hand on your belly with your inhalation, notice the natural pause, and then gently exhale, feeling your hand and your belly fall with the outbreath. Repeat this cycle of breathing in and out at least ten times, or for about two minutes. Allow yourself to observe how, without trying, your rate of breathing and heart rate slow down, your muscles relax, and your feeling of calm increases. Strive to do two minutes of belly breathing each morning and evening. Jot down what you observe in a journal.

Four-Square Breathing

"Four-square," or simply "square breathing," is another simple technique designed to elicit the relaxation response. This, too, should be practiced for a few minutes, twice daily, and can also be used whenever you find yourself feeling stressed.

Four-Square Breathing Exercise

You can sit, once again, with your spine fairly straight and your feet flat against the floor, or you can stand. Put one hand on your lower abdomen to help you remember to expand your diaphragm more fully when inhaling. Inhale to the count of four . . . then pause for the count of four . . . exhale for four counts . . . and pause for four counts. Repeat this cycle several times. Try for two minutes. It may take a bit for you to get used to the structured inhalation, pausing, and exhalation, but this will become easier with practice. As with belly breathing, you should notice an increased feeling of calm after doing four-square breathing.

Progressive Muscle Relaxation

Progressive muscle relaxation, or PMR, involves alternating tightening and then releasing voluntary muscles from your toes all the way up to your face (or if you prefer, your face all the way down to your toes—the order is really up to you). Set aside about thirty minutes when you can remain undisturbed. Use common sense and avoid tensing areas where your pain is active. If the idea of tensing *any* muscles is an unpleasant one, you may wish to ignore the suggestions to tense them and instead just follow the suggestions to simply breathe into these areas. Rewrite this script to suit your preferences and your doctor's advice with regard to contracting muscles or not.

You may also want to record yourself or someone else reading the instructions that follow, so you can focus most of your attention on simply doing the PMR exercise. Read the script at a slow, relaxed pace, pausing between each part you tense and relax (or simply relax), and when you see an ellipsis (. . .).

ALERT

Although PMR is generally considered safe and appropriate for chronic pain patients, you may want to print out the script and show the tensing/stretching exercises to your doctor to make sure each is appropriate for you. You can always modify by simply sending the breath to any area that feels tight or tense rather than tensing or stretching a muscle group.

PMR Exercise

Setting aside thirty minutes or so where you can remain undisturbed, begin by sitting with your spine comfortably straight, legs uncrossed, and hands resting in your lap. You may wish to put a pillow behind your head and neck. Alternatively, you can do the exercise lying down, again with your ankles uncrossed and hands at your sides or gently resting on your belly. Breathe in through your nose, and out through your mouth. Allow your awareness to notice any areas of tightness or tension and, gently breathing, send the image or feeling of comfort there, using your breath to help you focus on the sensation of relaxation.

Bring your awareness to your toes, and the soles of your feet. On the inhalation, curl your toes and tense the soles of your feet for a few seconds. Imagine you are squeezing out any tension or stress. Exhale through your mouth, and relax your toes and feet. Enjoy the release this provides. . . . Breathe easily, and deeply. Next, on the inhalation, draw your feet and toes up toward your shins, feeling the stretch up the calf muscles. Hold for a few seconds . . . exhale and release. Tighten your calf muscles now, hold for a few seconds . . . and release on the exhale once again.

Move your awareness to your thigh muscles, your quadriceps in the front, and your hamstrings in the back. Breathe. Tighten the front of your thighs on the inhalation. . . . If you are lying down, you can do this by trying to straighten your legs. You'll feel the muscles pulling your kneecap upwards. If you are seated, you can tense these muscles by pushing your heels down onto the floor. . . . Exhale and release. Just notice how nice that feels, to release any tension. Tighten your hamstrings now, the backs of your thighs, which you can do by bending your knees and bringing your heels toward your butt, or you can simply tense these muscles. . . . Exhale, and release.

Now, bring your attention to your buttocks. Breathe. On the next inhalation, tighten your butt muscles, squeezing firmly. Hold for a few seconds, and release on the exhalation. Breathe. . . .

Noticing your abdominal muscles, on the inhalation, tense your belly for a few seconds. You can do this by pulling your belly button in and up. Breathe out, relaxing your abdomen. . . . Feel the calm spreading from your lower body, upwards.

Now, bring your awareness to the muscles of your back. If you are sitting, you can reach your arms out in front of you as you stretch your back by moving it backward, away from your hands. Allow your pelvis, your hips, to pull forward with your arms and shoulders, as you gently move the middle of your back toward the chair. Feel the stretch across the upper back and the lower back. Exhale, and once again, align your hips, back, and shoulders. Breathe. Gently arch your back, then shift side to side, with your right shoulder leaning toward your right hip, which will stretch your left side . . . and then reversing this stretch by moving your left shoulder gently toward your left hip. Breathe and release.

On the next inhalation, raise your shoulders toward your ears . . . breathe and hold for a few seconds. Release on the exhalation. Gently roll your shoulders backward, in a circle, enjoying the stretch. Release, and allow the tension to flow out with the breath.

Bringing your awareness to your arms, contract your biceps muscles by curling your arm toward you, bringing your right hand to your right shoulder, and your left hand to your left shoulder. Tense and hold for a few seconds . . . now, exhale and relax your hands back down. Feel the release in the biceps muscles. Breathe. Bringing your attention to your wrists and forearms, inhale and flex your wrists, first moving your hands back toward you, feeling the contraction in the front of your forearm . . . then breathing out and releasing. Then bend your wrists gently forward, feeling the contraction on the inside of your forearms, and the stretch up the front. Exhale and release. Enjoy the pleasant heaviness you may be feeling in your arms, your breathing naturally becoming slower and deeper.

Now, noticing your hands, on the inhalation, clench them into fists, imagining squeezing out any tension or tightness, any frustration. Becoming more aware of your own strength, which is greater than you have imagined. Release on the exhale, perhaps with a big sigh of relief. Breathe. On the next inhalation, stretch your fingers by spreading them wide, savoring the wonderful release this brings. Breathe out . . . and relax your hands.

Moving your attention now to your neck and face, gently tilt your head back, feeling the stretch up the front of your neck and below your chin. Breathe, and allow your chin to be level with the floor or your feet. Tilt your head forward now, feeling the stretch up the back of your neck and in the middle of your upper back. Imagine these muscle fibers unwinding, like a knot loosening and releasing. Breathe normally, and return your head to level.

Contract the muscles of your face now, scrunching your nose and squeezing your cheeks up toward your eyes, drawing your brows toward your nose. Breathe. Enjoy being able to make this silly face, and release any tension in this area. Exhale, and release. Take turns raising your eyebrows, holding, and releasing them, gently moving your jaw side-to-side, and relaxing, and then yawning and stretching your jaw and mouth open, exhaling, and releasing.

Take a few minutes and some easy breaths, allowing yourself to stay with the feeling of increasing comfort and peace in your body. If you like, you can do this exercise before bed to help you fall asleep. Otherwise, you can set a timer to gently help you re-alert after thirty or forty minutes from when you begin. When you are ready, you can take a few more deep cleansing breaths. Stretch as you need to, slowly open your eyes, perhaps have a sip of water, and return to your day.

Cognitive Distortions

Everyone has times when they view the world through a lens that makes things seem worse than they are. The problem is that cognitive distortions can worsen your mood because you will take these assessments of yourself, others, and the world in general as true if you are not aware of which ones you tend to use and when you are using them. And if your mood, self-esteem, or optimism for the present and future are compromised, you will be less likely to engage in behaviors that could make your life better.

As discussed in other sections of this book, catastrophizing is quite common in chronic pain. The following is an abbreviated list of cognitive distortions that can make pain management more difficult. Note or circle those you tend to engage in most frequently. If at first you conclude that you never or rarely use any of these, it may be worth asking a trusted friend or other loved one for her input:

- *Black-and-white*, or *dichotomous thinking*, is also known as "all or nothing" thinking. This distortion leaves you unable to see the vast middle ground and can fuel feelings of anger, resentment, hopelessness, anxiety, etc. "Everyone is ignorant about chronic pain" and "All pain medication is useless" are examples of black-and-white thinking.
- *Overgeneralizing* refers to concluding something negative about an entire category of something based on one or a few negative experiences. "Dieting just doesn't work for me" is an example of overgeneralizing, because it's possible that you have not found the right eating plan for you. Thinking, "All doctors are just in it for the money" after a bad experience with one doctor is another example.
- *Fortunetelling* involves predicting a negative future (in the absence of objective evidence, such as a definitive medical prognosis). It can be a negative prediction about something big, like, "My pain will get worse and I won't be able to leave home" or something smaller, like, "I'm not going to like my physical therapist."
- *Unfair comparisons* are exactly what they sound like—comparing yourself or your progress to that of other people without taking into account that everyone is different and has different innate abilities, different bodies, different circumstances, and perhaps different levels of support. "Harry was able to run a mile after one month in physical therapy, and I can't even do half of that yet." Often, the unfair comparison is followed with *should*s, such as, "And I should be able to do this by now."

FACT

"Mind reading" is another type of cognitive distortion that can make coping with pain even more challenging. Mind reading leads you to assume you know what others are thinking of you (and you'll believe others are judging you negatively). For example, mind reading can lead you to conclude that another person's silence is indicative of their not liking you, disapproving of you, or doubting the validity of your pain, even in the absence of any evidence to this effect.

- *Shoulds* involves judging or interpreting events in terms of what you believe they should be like, rather than dealing with them as they are. Shoulds typically leave you believing you or others are inadequate or inferior, and leave you feeling angry, resentful, or hopeless as a result. "I should be able to do the activities I used to, already" and "My partner should always understand what I'm going through" are common examples.

- *Discounting the positives* involves being unable to recognize or minimizing the things you have been able to do, or what has been going well, and focusing on or amplifying the negatives. Some examples are, "My pain has improved by 30 percent, but who cares? It's not completely gone yet" and "Great, I walked my kid to school today, but so what? That's what parents are supposed to do."

Working with Cognitive Distortions

Once you become aware of the cognitive distortions you are most likely to use, you can then keep track of the situational and emotional factors that often accompany or trigger them. Keeping a diary of your emotions, cognitive distortions, and triggering events can help you interrupt a pattern of thinking that may have felt automatic until now. You can then "examine the evidence" for or against dysfunctional thoughts. If there is objective evidence that they represent something true, you will at least know what you are really confronting and can decide how you want to handle the situation before you. If the evidence does not support these negative thoughts, they are by definition cognitive distortions, and it is worth seeking to change them so they stop getting in the way.

Over the course of the next week, fill in the following table when you notice yourself engaging in thoughts that may be cognitive distortions.

Date	Event/Trigger	Thought	Emotion	Cognitive Distortion
4/29/15	Unable to do all of PT exercises	The woman next to me has the same diagnosis and she is doing so much better	Shame, frustration	Unfair comparison

After one week, note which cognitive distortions are most common for you. Then examine and challenge the evidence regarding each dysfunctional thought. Following are some strategies for challenging beliefs and thoughts, even if you have previously just accepted them as true.

Tips for Challenging Cognitive Distortions

The following is a list of tips that will help you combat cognitive distortions:

- Ask, *"What is the evidence* that this is true?" For something to be fundamentally true, it must be true *all the time* for you. If you are "just not good" at PT, it implies you never have been or never will be. If you could complete your physical therapy exercises three weeks ago, and you make progress next week, this contradicts the idea that you can't do it, aren't good at it, etc.
- *Look for the gray areas or middle ground.* Related to number one, few things are truly black and white. For example, if your doctor is late or curt one day, you may conclude, "My doctor must not really care about me." Or if a partner seems unhelpful or frustrated recently, you might conclude, "He just doesn't get me" or "He doesn't love me now that I'm

in pain." When you notice thinking in absolutes, ask yourself, "Is there a middle ground that I'm overlooking?" Assessing this on a scale of 0 to 100, and given all you know about this person or situation, how likely is it that your all-or-nothing statement is true? Similarly, if the distortion has to do with your ability to do something, or your self-worth, it's especially important to ask yourself these questions before attaching firmly to a conclusion.

- *Reframe your understanding* of the situation. "Sometimes I have better days than others" is a more accurate statement than, "I'm just not good at—" or "I cannot do—" something.

- *Would you come to the same conclusion about someone else in your situation*? If it seems easier to find "good reasons" why someone else might experience the challenges you are experiencing, if you would come to a more positive conclusion about that person, or if you would make a different prediction for that person, you are likely using distorted logic with regard to your own abilities, worth, or progress.

- *Explore alternatives*. If you are distressed because your pain has been spiking more lately, and have concluded that this means something dire about your health, write down other reasons why you or someone in a similar situation could have a flare-up or spike. Examples could include that you need to revisit pacing, or that there has been some change with regard to emotional or physical triggers. Examples of the latter include temperature changes during the transition from one season to another, changes in eating, sleep, or exercise, changes to your medication regimen, increased stress at work or home, upcoming holidays, etc. Even positive changes, such as going on a much-anticipated vacation, can lead to increases in pain or fatigue. So it's important to consider alternatives.

- *Do a reality check*. Ask other people you trust for their honest take on your conclusion, and if they think it is a realistic one. Be prepared for whatever their answers are. Are their assessments similar to yours? Different?

- *Dare to consider the "Worst Case Scenario."* This technique works especially well if you tend to catastrophize and then find yourself even more anxious or depressed as a result. If the thing you fear were to happen (e.g., your physical condition worsens, a person you love is angry at you, or you conclude you truly made a mistake), how would you deal with the issue then? If you have trouble knowing what you would do, imagine what you would advise a friend to do. Remember, very few things are truly catastrophic, and you can create an action plan if the feared outcome happens. Until then, most likely you are better off using your time and energy for other things.

- When all else fails to shed new light on the distortion, *ask yourself the Four Key Questions*: "Do I believe in my heart that this true?" "Is this *always* true?" and "How do I know this (what is the evidence)?" Write down the answers to these questions. Now ask yourself, "What would it mean for me if this belief *was not* true?" This last question can liberate you from the prison of negative thinking and distress.

Creating Positive Change

As you probably have gathered by now, CBT can help you understand the thoughts, feelings, and behaviors related to chronic pain, and also can shed light on what may be fueling distress or getting in the way of your goal of feeling better. Relatedly, CBT is a terrific tool for changing habits—whether you want to change the frequency of a behavior, such as increasing exercise, or decrease saturated fat in your diet; adopt a new behavior, such as begin a regular practice of meditation; or stop doing something, such as when you want to quit smoking. Even though these examples are not directly related to pain, they certainly impact how you feel on a number of levels, and thus are important to your pain management program.

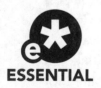

ESSENTIAL

Letting go of old habits and creating healthy new ones can seem daunting, but it is worth the effort and can help you manage pain and feel better overall. For a more in-depth, free report discussing how to create positive change, visit *http://blog.healthjourneys.com/update-from-belleruth/a-free-report-kicking-the-habit-ten-keys-to-positive-change.html*.

Because habits can become deeply engrained, so much so that you may feel like you are on "automatic pilot," it can feel daunting to try to change them. But these ten simple steps can help you to create positive changes in your life more easily:

1. **Identify the habit that you want to change.** Be very clear about what the new routine would ideally look like.

2. **Write down the pros and cons** of changing the habit or adopting a new one. Write down how you might address each potential con or barrier to making change. Understand that this list may evolve as you move forward in your process. If you have a hard time coming up with solutions, imagine what you would recommend to someone else.

3. **Craft a new routine.** Decide how you will work up to your goal. Usually this will involve breaking the larger goal into small, doable steps. As an example, if your goal is to drink eight glasses of water a day, and currently you are at four, adding one additional daily glass per week will make your goal feel easier to achieve than trying to make the shift all at once.

4. **Create a schedule.** Look at your calendar and decide by when you want to have implemented your new routine. Working backward, break this change into gradual steps. Do this regardless of whether the goal is to increase or decrease the behavior—the basic plan is the same. Each day, week, or month—depending on how long term your goal is—determine what progress will look like for you. Schedule these changes as you would any other important commitments.

5. **Decide on reward contingencies.** Contingencies help your brain change its expectations related to *how*, *when*, and *if* you will receive a reward. Specifically, contingencies set up a system whereby you can *only* have the reward *after* you have performed a specific behavior, or if it is performed at a certain time, etc. If you are trying to gradually cut down on, and then quit smoking, and your first cigarette of the day is usually at 8 A.M., week one of your program might be that you cannot have your first cigarette before 10 A.M. The following week, your first cigarette could not be before 11 A.M., and so forth. In this example, the target behavior (having a cigarette) is contingent upon it being a specific time, but not earlier. The contingency could just as well be a behavioral one, such as you cannot have that first cigarette until after you have completed your morning exercise routine.

6. **Add mindfulness to your toolbox.** Mindfulness will help you become much more aware of the chain of thoughts or events, feelings or cravings, and typical behaviors that make up the habit. Becoming more aware will enhance your power to change this chain.

7. **Create a psychological ritual.** Write down some of the worries related to making positive change. These might be thoughts such as, "I'm worried I will fail." Or, "I am afraid I will miss (insert habit)." You may also wish to write down what you dislike about the old tool, such as "Being dependent on (the habit)," or "Feeling bad about myself." Write down whatever comes to mind. *Breathe.* Visualize the relief you will feel when you have moved on from the habit. When you are ready, crumple the paper and discard it in the garbage outside your home. This is a symbolic way of removing from your immediate sphere the habit and the associated fears of letting go of it. Notice how it feels to release something that the healthiest part of you knows you no longer need.

8. **Engage in mental rehearsal.** Guided imagery and hypnosis are wonderful tools for changing habits, and recent studies have shown that hypnotically imagining something activates the brain in ways that are similar to actually *doing* it.

9. **"Experience" this change with as many senses as possible.** Using self-hypnosis or guided imagery, really "be" in your body as you engage in the new exercise regimen. Imagine how you will feel, and how your appearance or functioning will change, if these are relevant. Imagine how things will taste, smell, and sound, and allow yourself to enjoy "experiencing" already having reached your goal. The more you do this, the more vivid the benefits of making change will be for you, and the more powerful a tool your new routine will become.

10. **Strive to be compassionate, patient, and loving with yourself.** Doing so decreases distress and also helps you support yourself during a process of transition. Strive to do one simple, caring thing for yourself each day.

How to Find a CBT Therapist

The techniques described here are only a sampling of what you can learn and achieve in sessions with a qualified therapist. It may take a few tries to find the right fit for you with regard to a therapist's style of working, personality, and availability, but here are some tips for helping you find a provider who is trained in CBT and familiar with pain management:

- Ask your pain specialist for a referral. She may already know of someone who is appropriately trained and well regarded by both other professionals and pain patients like you.
- Contact your state psychological association and search for providers who indicate having expertise in both CBT and working with chronic pain. Most state associations have a member referral database that you can search online.
- Therapist referral sites, such as PsychologyToday.com and GoodTherapy .org will allow you to search for therapists who meet your individualized criteria, including location, therapeutic orientation, and whether or not they specialize in treating pain.
- If your local hospital or university medical center has a pain service, call and ask them which psychologists they typically recommend for treating chronic pain.

CHAPTER 14

Acupuncture

Acupuncture is an ancient, body-based therapy that belongs to the larger category of Traditional Chinese Medicine (TCM). Using long, thin needles, practitioners aim to balance the body's qi, or life force energy. Balanced qi leads to a healthier body, mind, and spirit. Acupuncture is one of the better-studied CAM therapies, both in general and for pain. It has been shown to help with several pain conditions, including back and neck pain, osteoarthritis, chronic headache, and shoulder pain.

What Is Acupuncture?

Acupuncture is a TCM technique that is believed to be at least two thousand years old. Acupuncture originated in China, but gained popularity in the Western world in the early 1970s. The classic TCM view of acupuncture is that vital or life force energy (qi) flows throughout the body via fourteen specific but invisible channels called meridians. Specific locations along these meridians, called acupoints, each correspond to different organs. (Subsequently, other styles of acupuncture have arisen that include additional meridians and acupoints, but the details of these systems are beyond the scope of this chapter.) Although TCM and the theories related to acupuncture are too complex to detail thoroughly here, what follows is a basic overview.

Acupuncture in the United States incorporates medical traditions from China, Japan, Korea, and other countries. The treatment is guided by the assumption that qi flows through the body, supporting proper function of all your organs and bodily functions, and also affecting your mood and thinking. Placing needles at various points along the meridians is thought to clear blockages or improve the flow of qi. It may be helpful to imagine the meridians as a network of invisible highways for your life force energy, and the hundreds of acupoints as important signposts that tell you where the energy may be blocked, and thus where to intervene.

The Acupuncture Session

There are now many different styles of acupuncture; thus, acupuncturists' assessments and needle placement will vary somewhat. In general, however, at your first session the provider will take a detailed history of your primary complaint, as well as ask you other questions about your health. Even if you seek treatment for migraine pain, your acupuncturist will ask you questions about things such as the quality of your sleep, diet, appetite, digestion, skin, allergies, menstrual cycle (if you are a woman), and so forth. It's not uncommon for an acupuncturist to then examine your tongue to observe its color and type of coating and also take your pulse multiple times, with minor adjustments in position and pressure, on both your wrists.

Then, while you are either normally clothed or wearing a paper gown or robe (such as you might during a medical doctor's examination), you will lie comfortably on a massage table while the acupuncturist applies alcohol swabs to the areas where she will place needles. She will then insert sterile, very fine, stainless steel acupuncture needles at various places on your body, which can include your scalp, face, ears, chest, back, arms, legs, feet, or midsection. After the needles have been properly placed, your acupuncturist will then gently twirl or otherwise manipulate the needles to move and balance your qi. You may not feel much of anything when the needles are inserted or manipulated, or you may feel a mild to moderate pinching or "electrical" sensation. Most people find acupuncture tolerable and the sessions overall very relaxing.

After the needles have been inserted, it takes about thirty minutes for acupuncture to reach its full potential for decreasing pain. Your acupuncturist will leave the room so you can rest quietly. During this time, you can benefit additionally from mindfully bringing your awareness to your breath, or engaging in another type of relaxation. You will be most comfortable if you limit movement during this period, as the needles can cause mild, transient discomfort if you flex your muscles while shifting position.

Although the frequency of treatment will vary depending on your health issues and your provider's recommendation, typically, sessions are weekly but not more than twice weekly. It may take five or six weeks of treatments for you to determine if acupuncture is helpful for you.

FACT

According to TCM, your acupuncturist may place needles close to, far from, or both near and far from the area you hope to balance. Don't be surprised if you seek treatment for indigestion and have needles placed on your abdomen, in the web of your hand, and on top of your foot!

What Does the Science Say?

A good deal of research has been conducted on acupuncture. A recent study of acupuncture found that it resulted in greater pain relief than sham (fake) acupuncture and standard care alone. Other studies have found that acupuncture activates several areas of the brain involved in movement, sensing touch, decision-making, regulating emotions, and more. Acupuncture also appears to affect levels of neurotransmitters (brain chemicals) involved in mood and pain. Furthermore, acupuncture appears to impact the release of endogenous opioids and enkephalins, or the brain's and CNS's natural pain medicines.

FACT

In 1971, an American journalist suffered an attack of appendicitis while on assignment in China. He had an emergency appendectomy, and post-operatively received acupuncture to alleviate significant abdominal discomfort and distension. His story made national news, and is available here: *http://acupunctureworldheadquarters.com/1971acupuncture.pdf*.

In China, acupuncture has been used with conventional anesthesia in an effort to reduce the anesthetic medication needed during surgery. At present, the evidence is not yet sufficient to recommend decreasing anesthesia during surgery across the board; however, there is data showing that acupuncture performed during surgery can reduce postoperative pain, decrease the number of postoperative pain medications, and lead to shorter hospital stays.

It's important to note that acupuncture can probably be helpful for most, but not all people. In those for whom it works, acupuncture can raise the pain threshold (i.e., decrease sensitivity to pain). As of this writing, the pain conditions for which there is the most evidence that acupuncture can help are low-back pain, neck pain, and osteoarthritis/knee pain. Acupuncture also may help reduce the frequency of tension headaches and prevent migraine headaches.

Although, to date, the best evidence for acupuncture is as a treatment for pain relief, there are many other conditions for which people seek acupuncture treatments, and for which there is likely benefit. Among these are allergies, fatigue, indigestion, nausea, vomiting, insomnia, infertility, menstrual irregularities, and other issues.

Terri's Tongue Told the Tale

Terri was working part-time as a personal trainer in addition to her desk job. Her hip joints and back and neck muscles were already tight from working at a computer all day. When, during a personal training session, Terri lifted a weight that was too heavy for her, Terri's back and neck pain went from mild to stabbing, intense discomfort. Her sleep and fatigue, which were normally problematic, worsened significantly. Terri tried to manage her fatigue with extra cups of coffee, but this caused heartburn without making her feel fully alert. It became harder to stay awake and concentrate at her desk job, and her limited mobility at the gym was getting in the way of training clients.

Terri's doctor offered her a muscle relaxant and a narcotic pain medicine, but she was conflicted about taking them. A friend had recommended acupuncture, and Terri decided to give it a try. At the initial appointment, a Chinese-trained medical doctor who was also a licensed acupuncturist took a detailed medical history, checked Terri's pulses, and looked carefully at Terri's tongue.

"Why are you examining my *tongue*?" Terri asked. "I mean, what does that have to do with my pain?"

Dr. Deng told her, "The coating, size, color, and shape of the tongue can tell me something about your health. Your tongue tells me you have indigestion. So does the state of your hair and nails. Am I correct?"

Terri was stunned by this observation, as she had experienced IBS since adolescence. Her high coffee consumption further aggravated this condition. Terri had neglected to tell Dr. Deng about this issue as she thought it irrelevant to the pain condition she was hoping he could treat.

Continuing his exam, Dr. Deng also correctly noted Terri's sinusitis. They discussed her fatigue, as well as the worry that was keeping her up at night. Dr. Deng said he would strive to address all of these with TCM, especially acupuncture and acupressure massage. He also made suggestions about proper diet and the importance of making mealtime sacred, to help Terri's body better digest her food. Although Terri was initially skeptical and found the acupressure very different from the Swedish massages she had tried previously, after having had her eighth weekly session and making the lifestyle changes Dr. Deng had recommended, she had an interesting realization.

"It was the strangest thing. One day, I was walking into work and I realized I had passed my usual coffee shop—*without* stopping to get my normal large coffee—the first of the four I had been having per day. I almost turned around to get it, but I was struck by the fact that I felt so much better—less tired and in less pain than I had been in months. It actually took me a while to realize that my symptoms had quieted down and that my body felt pretty good. Then I just felt giddy."

Many acupuncturists, if they are well trained in TCM, will take a whole-person approach to health. It's common for them to make dietary and other lifestyle recommendations. Your acupuncturist may also recommend the use of Chinese herbs for a variety of health issues.

ALERT

Use Chinese herbal remedies with caution, particularly if they are imported from overseas. Herbal preparations may contain contaminants, and the ingredients are not standardized—both of which can lead to harm. Always discuss herbal remedies with your physician to avoid possible herb-drug interactions.

Types of Acupuncture

Although your acupuncturist may insert and manipulate the needles as described, he may also apply heat or use mild electrical stimulation, which is referred to as electroacupuncture. In many acupuncture studies, electroacupuncture is used because it is easier to standardize the degree of stimulation electrically than by manually manipulating needles.

Acupressure is technically a type of massage because the acupoints are stimulated by the practitioner's hands and fingers, rather than via insertion of needles. The principle behind this technique is that, like acupuncture, acupressure moves and balances qi. Practitioners should be licensed or certified massage therapists who are also trained specifically in acupuncture or in Asian bodywork.

Acupressure is different from other types of massage in that the practitioner may use his elbows or feet in addition to using his hands and fingers to apply more forceful pressure where needed, and acupressure may be combined with acupuncture or other TCM therapies. Depending on the practitioner and the amount of pressure she applies, acupressure can feel very intense and somewhat uncomfortable if you have significant muscle imbalances or soreness. It's important to discuss painful areas with your massage therapist ahead of time and maintain clear communication if the pressure feels too intense for you.

ALERT

Acupuncture needles should be sterile and their packaging opened just before your acupuncturist places them on the acupoints related to your issues. If your acupuncturist retrieves needles from a jar of what appears to be alcohol, rather than from a sealed package, do not proceed with the session.

Training of Acupuncturists

As of this writing, each state has its own criteria for credentialing; some states do not regulate acupuncture at all. To find out the requirements to practice acupuncture in a particular state, visit *www.acufinder.com/Acupuncture+Laws*.

Currently, forty-three states plus the District of Columbia require that acupuncturists have been certified by the National Certification Commission for Acupuncture and Oriental Medicine (NCCAOM). This certification results in the practitioner becoming a Diplomate of Acupuncture. A Diplomate of Acupuncture completes three to four academic years of education at the master's degree level in an acupuncture program accredited by the Accreditation Commission for Acupuncture and Oriental Medicine (ACAOM). ACAOM is the only accrediting body recognized by the United States Department of Education as the authority for quality education and training in acupuncture and Oriental medicine.

As an alternative to being certified by NCCAOM, some states require a passing score on the NCCAOM certification examinations. Other states require that an acupuncturist be a licensed health professional.

How to Find a Qualified Acupuncturist

In addition to NCCAOM certification and licensure, some state regulatory boards award the designation of licensed acupuncturist (L.Ac.).

Alternatively, your doctor, nurse, or chiropractor can become certified to provide acupuncture. A significant "pro" of seeing a medical provider for acupuncture is that they are trained in the standards, ethics, and practice of Western medicine. The American Academy of Medical Acupuncture requires a minimum of 220 hours of related training and a medical, dental, veterinary, or nursing license to become an affiliate member. To become a full member, one must also have been practicing acupuncture for at least five years and have published or taught related to acupuncture.

From a TCM perspective, a "con" of seeing a medical acupuncturist is that medical acupuncturists receive considerably fewer hours of training in TCM compared to someone who has received master's level training in these CAM areas. Ultimately, you will want to consider how many providers you have the time and financial resources to see. If your physician or nurse can evaluate and treat your pain from both a Western and acupuncture perspective, this may be very appealing.

If you are hoping to have an in-depth evaluation and acupuncture treatment based primarily or solely on TCM, and you can afford to have separate conventional and CAM providers, then a well-trained, nonmedical acupuncturist may be a better fit. If you choose treatment with a nonmedical acupuncturist, it is worth finding one who will communicate and collaborate with your conventional medical team. Similarly, it is helpful if your medical team is receptive to your use of acupuncture and also willing to maintain open lines of communication among providers.

Insurance Coverage

Because acupuncture has a growing body of research supporting its effectiveness, many insurance companies now offer some form of coverage or reimbursement for acupuncture, particularly if it is used to treat pain. Contact your insurer to learn whether this service is covered and what your out-of-pocket expenses will be. Inquire if coverage varies depending on whether the acupuncture is provided by a non-medical versus a physician acupuncturist.

Here are some tips for deciding whether to pursue acupuncture if your insurance does not cover it:

- Ask your healthcare provider if she recommends a particular acupuncturist and research other credentialed acupuncturists in your area
- Determine how much you can realistically afford to spend out of pocket each week

- Contact credentialed practitioners near you and inquire about their fees for both the consultation and individual sessions
- Assume you will need a minimum of six weekly sessions before you see a benefit from acupuncture, and multiply your weekly budget by this number to realistically assess your acupuncture expenses
- If the fees for reputable acupuncturists exceed what you can afford, ask practitioners if they offer a sliding scale

ESSENTIAL

It's important to find an acupuncturist who is properly trained and credentialed. To find a nonmedical but master's level acupuncturist, visit *http://mx.nccaom.org/FindAPractitioner.aspx*. To find a medical or health professional who is a credentialed acupuncturist, visit *www.medicalacupuncture.org/FindanAcupuncturist.aspx*.

CHAPTER 15

Hands-On Treatments

Long before there were formalized touch therapies, people used their hands to help others increase comfort and relaxation, and mobilize their innate abilities to heal. Chiropractic, osteopathic medicine, and massage are just a few of the therapeutic approaches that draw upon touch and the human connection to help ease pain and foster greater well-being. Although there is some overlap among these three healing systems, each has a unique approach to correcting structural imbalances, improving circulation, and easing discomfort.

Chiropractic

Chiropractic was formally established as a healthcare discipline in the late 1800s. According to the American Chiropractic Association, chiropractic focuses on disorders of the musculoskeletal system and the nervous system, as well as on the effects of these disorders on other areas of the body, and your health in general. Chiropractic care is used most often to treat neuromusculoskeletal complaints, including but not limited to back pain, neck pain, pain in the joints of the arms or legs, and headaches. One of the major principles of chiropractic has been the idea of treating the whole person, rather than treating the symptomatic part alone. Chiropractic also assumes that the body has potential for self-healing.

FACT

According to the NCCIH, approximately 4 million people will use chiropractic for back pain in a given year. A recent survey by Consumer Reports found that consumers felt chiropractic care was more beneficial than other therapies in the treatment of back pain.

A core feature of chiropractic is to assess and treat issues related to your spine via spinal manipulation (also known as adjustments), but your treatment may also include other therapies such as massage, electrical or ultrasound stimulation, recommendations for exercise and stretching, dietary suggestions and nutritional supplements. If he thinks it is necessary, the chiropractor may order X-rays or other imaging. Based on the results of your physical exam and any diagnostic findings, your chiropractor may adjust your spine either manually or by using an instrument called an activator. Adjustments move joints through their full range of motion and thereby realign and restore balance to an area.

Who Provides Chiropractic Care?

Chiropractors attend nationally accredited, four-year graduate training programs and upon completion receive a Doctor of Chiropractic (DC) degree. Chiropractic education includes courses in the biomedical sciences, public health, and research methods, as well as direct experience in providing clinical care. Although they cannot prescribe medications, chiropractors are considered to be physician-level providers in most states and by Medicare, Medicaid, and other federal programs. As such, in most states, chiropractors can order X-rays and in some cases, or with special training, they can perform more complex imaging such as MRIs, ultrasounds, and CT scans.

In order to become licensed, chiropractors must pass a series of four national board exams. Some chiropractors also complete postgraduate residencies in order to undergo additional, specialized training in areas such as orthopedics, neurology, or radiology. For more information on the training of chiropractors, visit *www.acatoday.org.*

FACT

The American College of Physicians and the American Pain Society issued a joint recommendation stating that for patients who do not improve with self-care options, clinicians should consider adding non-medical treatments such as chiropractic, massage, yoga, acupuncture, CBT, and relaxation.

The Chiropractic Consultation

As with other healthcare providers, at your consultation a chiropractor will typically ask about the issue you hope to resolve. She will then take a health history and perform a physical examination. Even if you present for a focused pain issue, such as back or neck pain, the chiropractor will likely ask you about your health overall, including your digestion, sleep, mood, and other areas of functioning. The chiropractor will then develop a treatment plan specific to your current health and goals. The American Chiropractic Association has a brief video describing what you can expect from your visit. You can view it here: *www.youtube.com/watch?v=yMqvjEX0mjU &feature=youtu.be.*

Chiropractic tends to value an integrative approach, and if it appears this may be helpful, your chiropractor may refer you for massage, energy work, acupuncture, or another CAM therapy. To find a chiropractor near you, visit *www.acatoday.org.*

According to the National Health Interview Survey, more than 18 million adults and nearly 2 million children have received chiropractic or osteopathic manipulation in the past year. Furthermore, 66 percent of people using chiropractic for back pain said it had "great benefit."

What the Science Says about Chiropractic

According to the NCCIH, in addition to being possibly helpful for low-back pain, spinal manipulation may be helpful for migraines as well as for headaches related to problems in the cervical spine. Chiropractic also appears to be helpful for upper and lower extremity joint conditions and whiplash. It is not clear whether chiropractic is helpful for fibromyalgia, mid-back pain, premenstrual syndrome, sciatica, or temporomandibular joint disorder.

Overall, chiropractic appears to be safe, although side effects can include transient headaches, fatigue, or discomfort. Serious complications are rare, and can include developing a pinched nerve or worsening of a herniated disc.

The NCCIH has a video summarizing the research on chiropractic for back pain. You can view it here: *www.youtube.com/watch?v=J5sng4aSvKI.*

Osteopathic Medicine

Osteopathic medicine (OM) was founded in the late 1800s by a medical doctor who believed that medicine should focus on prevention, be holistic, and work with the body's own ability to heal. OM involves diagnosis and manipulation of the spine, bones, and muscles. This may involve stretching or applying pressure to the muscles, thrusts or force applied against a joint to restore range of motion, techniques to encourage lymphatic drainage (to eliminate toxins from the body), and gently manipulating the cranium (bones of the skull), among others.

Training of Osteopathic Physicians

According to the American Osteopathic Association, to become an osteopathic physician an individual must graduate from an osteopathic medical school accredited by the American Osteopathic Association's Commission on Osteopathic College Accreditation. This accreditation is recognized by the U.S. Department of Education. As with MD programs, the curriculum at osteopathic medical schools consists of four years of study and emphasizes preventive medicine and comprehensive patient care. Thus, many osteopathic physicians become primary care or family practice doctors. Osteopathic physicians also undergo postgraduate training and are licensed by the same state licensing boards as MDs.

The training of DOs, as osteopathic physicians are also called, is essentially equivalent to that of medical doctors, with the addition of training in the musculoskeletal system and *osteopathic manipulative treatment (OMT)*. Osteopathic physicians can thus do everything an MD can do, from prescribing and monitoring medications, to ordering diagnostic work-ups, to performing surgery. OMT emphasizes using the hands to diagnose and treat illness and injury, but your DO may also incorporate more conventional therapies with OMT (drugs, surgery, etc.) if this is warranted.

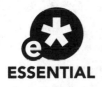

ESSENTIAL

A new survey by the American Osteopathic Association found that nine in ten office workers would be willing to do stretches or other exercises at work to prevent and relieve pain. Doing even a minute of stretching every hour can help you reduce or prevent pain.

Like chiropractic, OM also emphasizes a whole-person approach to healing. A principle of OM is that musculoskeletal restrictions that cause pain can either be a result or a source of physical dysfunction and disease. Sometimes health issues may be caused by restriction of a single joint; other times they are related to changes in posture, mobility, inflammation, and other factors.

What the Science Says about Osteopathic Manipulation

To date, most of the research on manual therapies for pain has been on physical therapy, chiropractic, or massage, rather than on OMT specifically.

The NCCIH also addresses OMT and chiropractic together in their overview, although the therapies are not identical. These therapies are likely discussed together because both employ the use of spinal manipulative therapy (SMT).

FACT

SMT is one of the most investigated CAM therapies, with the majority of studies looking at the effects of SMT on back pain, neck pain, and headaches secondary to cervical spine issues. More research is needed, but the data suggest SMT may decrease pain severity and increase the number of pain-free days.

In general, spinal manipulation has been shown to be helpful for low back and neck pain, and appears promising for headache pain. One study of patients with acute back pain found that OMT resulted in an equal improvement in pain to standard medical therapy, and the OMT group required fewer physical therapy visits and significantly less pain medication, anti-inflammatory drugs, and muscle relaxants. Another study of patients with sub-acute (lasting two-to-twelve weeks) spine pain found that adding three sessions of osteopathic manipulation improved short-term physical symptoms and longer term psychological ones. A study of patients with tension-type headaches found that OMT resulted in reduced headache frequency.

In general, OMT is considered safe and effective when done by a trained DO. Reports of serious complications are rare. Side effects include muscle soreness, temporary increases in pain following more vigorous manipulation, lightheadedness, and headache. To learn more about OM, visit *www.osteopathic.org/Pages/default.aspx.*

FACT

Nearly two in three office workers report being in pain. Sitting at a desk can cause poor posture, neck and back pain, and eye strain.
For a helpful infographic on common sources of pain at work, visit *www.osteopathic.org/osteopathic-health/about-your-health/health-conditions-library/pain/Documents/pain-and-productivity-infographic.pdf.*

To summarize, osteopathic manipulation is considered helpful for low back pain and may also be helpful for other pain conditions, including tension-type headache and migraines. Because DOs are fully licensed physicians in every state, they can provide both OMT and conventional medical treatment, and their services should be covered by insurance. As always, verify with your insurance carrier if the provider you wish to see is in-network or, if not, what your out-of-network costs would be.

To find an osteopathic physician near you, visit *www.osteopathic.org/ osteopathic-health/Pages/find-a-do-search.aspx*.

Massage

Massage is thought to be one of the oldest forms of hands-on healing, probably for good reason. As you learned in the chapter on the physiology of pain, nonpainful touch can help close the pain gate. Although any compassionate touch will likely feel healing and comforting, therapeutic massage can also help stretch tight muscles, loosen painful knots, and improve circulation. Massage can quite easily be paired with other CAM therapies, such as energy healing and the use of aromatherapy oils and lotions.

Massage, not surprisingly, is one of the most popular forms of CAM used by adults in the United States. The term massage is a very broad one, however. There are more varieties of massage than can be listed here, but examples include Swedish, shiatsu, deep tissue, lymphatic drainage, Thai, sports, and acupressure massage. Some types of massage, like acupressure, purport to move energy within the body. And many massage therapists combine techniques, tailoring them to the needs of the individual client. Although types of massage may vary significantly, in general, massage is intended to promote comfort, improve physical functioning in some way, and support the body's own tendency to self-heal.

The Massage Appointment

Many massage therapists will either have you fill out paperwork beforehand or ask you questions about any pain or injuries you may have, allergies, or other issues that may be important to know before commencing treatment. In order to make it easier to perform the massage and to protect your clothing from any lotions or oils that are used, you will often be asked to undress to your underwear and lie underneath a sheet or blanket on a massage table, in a room that is dimly lit to encourage relaxation. There may be soothing music playing in the background, as well.

The massage therapist will knead, stretch, press on, or otherwise work on most of your muscle groups, from your head to your toes, avoiding your breasts and genital areas. Many will massage the gluteal muscles (your butt), as these tend to hold tension and can become painful or uncomfortable. If there is any area that you prefer the therapist not touch, however, either because of pain or personal preference, it is absolutely important and appropriate to let her know this (and you will not be the first person to do so). Once the massage is complete, your therapist will probably put a hand gently on your back and quietly inform you that the session has ended.

Some types of massage, such as shiatsu, are done without the use of oils or lotions, and with you remaining fully clothed. In addition, some types of bodywork involve passively stretching your muscles in a way that may feel similar to physical therapy.

FACT

According to the 2007 NHIS, nearly 33 percent of those with pain or neurological issues, compared to 21 percent of those without those conditions, reported using CAM because of their healthcare provider's recommendation.

Credentialing of Massage Therapists

Most states regulate the massage therapy profession. Depending on the state, this could be in the form of a license, registration, or certification. Statewide massage therapy regulations will define the minimum massage therapy-training requirement. Most states require a minimum of 500 hours of training, but some states, such as New York, require 1,000 hours. Massage education should include supervised, in-class initial massage therapy training, including the study of anatomy and physiology, the theory and practice of massage therapy, and other subjects.

Although not required, massage therapists may choose to become board certified in massage therapy. The board certification is administered by the National Certification Board for Therapeutic Massage & Bodywork (NCBTMB). Individuals who meet standards of education, training, and experience, and pass the examination are entitled to use the designation Board Certified in Therapeutic Massage and Bodywork, and its initials, BCTMB.

To learn more about the regulations in your state, visit *www .amtamassage.org/regulation/stateRegulations.html*. To search for a massage therapist near you, including one who is trained in a specific technique, visit *www.amtamassage.org*.

Data from the NHIS found that compared to those not in pain, those with pain or neurological conditions were more likely to report that they used CAM because conventional treatment did not work and was too expensive.

What the Science Says about Massage

There are inherent challenges to evaluating the effects of therapeutic massage. In a society where in-person interactions, and therefore touch, have become more rare, the introduction of any form of compassionate touch has the potential to enhance relaxation or comfort—and in essence, be healing. That aside, there have been numerous studies of massage therapy and there is some evidence that massage is helpful for pain.

For example, a 2013 study of in-home massage for patients with metastatic cancer found that even receiving two to three massages was linked to significantly improved quality of life and a trend toward improvements in pain and sleep. The benefits did not last beyond the one-week follow-up, but there were also no negative effects associated with receiving massage.

Another study of patients who had rheumatoid arthritis found that a month of once-weekly arm and shoulder massage plus daily self-massage was linked to less pain and greater perceived grip strength and greater range of motion in the wrist and large upper joints (elbows and shoulders).

Moderate-pressure massage was linked to greater benefits than light-pressure massage.

An NCCIH-funded study found that multiple sixty-minute massages per week were more effective than fewer or shorter sessions for people with chronic neck pain, suggesting that several hour-long massages per week may be the best dose for people with this condition.

Massage has also been found to have modest, short-term benefits for fibromyalgia symptoms. And another NCCIH-funded study with patients who had advanced cancer and moderate-to-severe pain found that both massage and simple touch were linked to significant improvements in pain relief, physical and emotional distress, and quality of life. The effects were greater with massage.

In summary, massage appears to be helpful for several types of musculoskeletal pain, is generally considered safe, and has shown benefits with regard to reducing stress, increasing relaxation, and improving quality of life, including in patients who are medically ill. Massage may also improve range of motion and facilitate better sleep. Moderate pressure touch may have a greater benefit than light touch, and the benefits of receiving massage appear to increase with greater frequency of treatment (i.e., a few times per week rather than once weekly or less).

ALERT

Although generally safe, avoid massaging areas near a cancerous tumor, areas that are healing from surgery or radiation, areas that are infected or inflamed, areas where you have nerve pain, or areas near varicose veins. If you are pregnant, consult your doctor before pursuing massage, and inform your massage therapist of any health issues.

Self-Massage Techniques

Although you will not be able to reach every tense area as well as a massage therapist can, what follows are a few examples of self-massage that you may wish to try. Remember to breathe slowly and deeply to enhance relaxation, and avoid any position that causes discomfort or strain.

If you are unsure of whether it is safe to massage a specific area, consult with your doctor or physical therapist first. They will also be able to tell you about other techniques you can practice for pain relief, and may be able to refer you to a massage therapist who is experienced at working with chronic pain.

- *Shoulder and back massage*—bend your right arm, and gently lift it by the elbow until your hand can easily reach the left shoulder. Using the first two fingers of your right hand, gently but firmly press and massage any areas that are tight or tense, from your shoulder up to where your shoulder meets your neck, holding for a few seconds before moving on to the next area. If you can reach the middle of your upper back, on either side of your spine, you can gently massage this area as well. Switch sides and repeat.
- *Scalp massage*—bring both hands to the front of your scalp, thumbs above your temples and pinkies on your scalp, above your forehead, fingers comfortably spread. Gently move your hands so your fingers make small circles, gradually moving your hands back across your scalp. Let the feeling of comfort guide your hands.
- *Foot massage*—sitting comfortably in a chair, bend your right knee to bring your right foot to rest either on the chair, facing your left knee, or rest your foot on your left knee if this is comfortable. Massage the heel of your foot with your thumbs by making small, circular movements. Adjust the pressure so that it is sufficiently firm, but not so much that it causes discomfort. Experiment with the amount of pressure that feels most soothing. Continue making small circles with your thumbs, moving them down your foot toward your toes and massaging the fleshy footpad just below your toes. Then, hold each individual toe, one by one massaging and then moving each toe in a circular motion, first clockwise and then counterclockwise. If you like, you can use an aromatherapy oil or lotion to enhance the feeling of relaxation.

CHAPTER 16

Healing Power of the Senses

The use of both music and pleasant scents to enhance health and well-being dates back thousands of years. Music can set the tone for relaxation, inspire you to move your body, and stimulate creativity, and music therapy has more recently emerged as a formal discipline. Essential oils were extracted from herbs and flowers to create medicines and perfumes, to scent one's home, and to anoint the ill. Today, both aromatherapy and music can be easily combined with many CAM therapies, including massage, energy healing, hypnosis, meditation, and others to enhance relaxation and foster a sense of ease.

Music Therapy

According to the American Music Therapy Association, music therapy is an established health profession in which music is used to address the physical, emotional, cognitive, and social needs of individuals. After meeting with a client and discussing his current concerns and goals for treatment, a music therapist will create a program that can include composing music, singing, movement, and active listening. Music therapy also aims to provide an alternate means of communication for those who find it difficult to express themselves in words.

What the Science Says

A growing number of studies have examined whether music therapy is useful for pain management. Overall, it appears music can help both with easing pain and reducing distress. The analgesic effect of music has been demonstrated with both acute and chronic pain, as well as on pain induced in the laboratory setting.

Music has also been found to have other benefits in addition to pain relief. As with many CAM therapies, the quality of the research has been variable, and better-designed studies will shed more light on how music therapy works and who is most likely to benefit from which types of music. In general, however, music is considered a safe intervention and appeals to most people. Listening to music that one enjoys seems to be particularly helpful with regard to both distracting from pain and reducing distress. Music has even been shown to improve cognitive performance.

Music and Pain

What follows is necessarily a brief overview of the research on music and pain, but will give you a good idea of how music might help with a variety of concerns. For example, a 2014 review of CAM therapies looked at the results of five studies of music as a tool for managing pain. The conclusion was that music was effective for controlling pain in patients with cancer, osteoarthritis, chronic nonmalignant pain, and patients with lumbar pain, fibromyalgia, inflammatory disease, or a neurological disease.

A small, 2010 study with hospitalized burn patients found that music therapy, which included using music-based imagery and active listening, reduced pain, anxiety, and muscle tension associated with dressing changes.

Another small study looked at the impact of music on pain during physical therapy, and found that listening to music during PT led to significant decreases in pain as compared to PT without music. And yet another small study with Turkish patients who were hospitalized with neuropathic pain found that listening to classical Turkish music for one hour reduced pain. This benefit increased between the thirty- and sixty-minute marks, suggesting a greater benefit from a larger "dose."

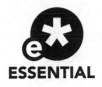

ESSENTIAL

The research suggests that listening to music you would rate as "pleasant" and that generates positive emotions is linked to reduced pain, anger, and anxiety, whereas listening to "unpleasant" music does not improve any of these symptoms.

In addition to these findings, music has been shown to reduce pain and improve functional mobility in patients with fibromyalgia. And another study examining the effect of both music engagement (how absorbed one can become in listening) and trait anxiety (how anxious you tend to be in general) predicted how well listening to music could reduce pain. Specifically, those who tended to be more anxious as a rule, and those who are able to become more deeply absorbed in music listening, experienced the greatest benefits.

To summarize, music may help with pain by:

- Increasing pleasant emotion
- Stimulating the brain's reward centers (as described in the next section)
- Blocking pain in the spinal cord before it reaches your brain
- Serving as a pleasant distraction

Key factors that influence how likely you are to benefit from music include:

- The more you like your musical selection, and the more engaged you are in listening, the more likely the music is to decrease pain perception
- Pleasant-sounding music is typically more effective than unpleasant-sounding, or discordant music
- The effect of listening to music appears to increase over the course of a session of listening
- People who tend to be anxious and can easily become absorbed in music may see an even greater benefit
- Music seems to help with a variety of different pain conditions and also can reduce pain that is deliberately generated in the laboratory setting

Music and the Brain

Modern technology has shed new light on how music affects the brain and body. It has also revealed how music may have other benefits beyond reducing pain, for both medically ill and healthy individuals.

Recent research has revealed that the pleasure generated by music activates the brain's reward system and increases the amount of the neurotransmitter dopamine. Relatedly, music has been shown to generate activity in emotion-processing areas of the brain, and it is generally accepted that musical selections can influence emotional states. In addition, music can cause changes in heart rate, blood pressure, respiration rate, and other bodily functions depending on the type of emotion that a particular musical selection generates.

Beyond the simple pleasure of listening, music is processed by a number of different areas of the brain, including ones involved in spoken language. In fact, a number of studies have shown temporary cognitive benefits associated with listening to pleasant music, including improved information-processing speed, reasoning, attention and memory, and creativity. Music therapy has also helped people who have had strokes to improve their gait, mood, speech, and social interactions. Understanding the impact of music on cognitive ability may be especially important for those who have noticed cognitive changes due to aging, illness, or medication.

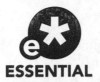

In some studies, verbal material that was presented in a musical context was learned and recalled better than spoken verbal material. So, next time you need to memorize something, whether your grocery list or material for an upcoming exam, set it to your favorite tune!

Music Therapy and Visual Processing

Visual neglect is the inability to recognize objects in part of the visual field due to lesions (or damage) in the brain's visual cortex. Specifically, a lesion in one hemisphere produces neglect in the opposite visual field. In other words, a stroke in the left visual cortex could result in one being unable to recognize objects in the right visual field, and vice versa.

In one study of stroke patients experiencing visual neglect, listening to pleasant music resulted in both better mood and a significant improvement in their ability to describe the color and shape of geometric objects presented via computer. No such effects were observed when participants sat in silence or when they were presented with music that they did not like.

Further examination with functional magnetic resonance imaging (fMRI) confirmed that listening to pleasant music activated a number of different brain areas, including those involved in visual processing.

Memory, Attention, and Mood

In another study with people who had recently experienced a stroke, listening to music was linked to greater recovery of verbal memory and focused attention in the music group versus listening to an audiobook or sitting in silence. Furthermore, the music group participants had significantly less depression and confusion than those in the no-intervention group. This benefit was seen within the first three months of listening.

Listening to music also helped these stroke patients increase their motor activity. Preliminary imaging results suggest that listening to music following a stroke may result in measurable changes to both the structure and function of the brain. In summary, music may reduce the negative effects of stress on the brain and body, improve cognitive function and mood, and impact brain chemicals that play a role in recovery.

Music and Medication Needs

A 2006 Cochrane review of the research on music and pain concluded that music did, in fact, result in reductions in pain versus not listening to music, and that listening to music resulted in roughly a 15–18 percent decrease in morphine use after surgery. The review also found that listening to music during a painful procedure resulted in a trend toward lower pain medication requirements than not listening to music. The authors concluded that listening to music does reduce pain intensity and opioid pain medication requirements, but that the amount of the reduction is small.

Although there is still more to learn about how and why music helps in so many ways, it is worth making time for music to move your body, enhance comfort, engage your mind, and soothe your soul.

Training of Music Therapists

Music therapists must have completed either a bachelor's- or master's-level music therapy curriculum and then passed a national examination. Music therapists who successfully complete the examination hold the credential Music Therapist, Board Certified (MT-BC). To verify an individual's certification credentials, visit *http://cbmt.org*. Other designations include: RMT (Registered Music Therapist), CMT (Certified Music Therapist), and ACMT (Advanced Certified Music Therapist). While new RMT, CMT, and ACMT designations are no longer awarded, those who have received and continue to maintain them are qualified to practice music therapy.

Adding Music to Your Daily Life

Given the research on music's potential to reduce pain and distress, improve cognition and functioning, as well as its broad appeal, it's worth adding music to your pain management plan. Whether you decide to work with a music therapist or want to begin by incorporating music on your own is up to you. What follows are some simple and effective strategies for adding music into your daily life:

- Select music that you like and that tends to enhance positive mood for you
- Keep notes about which songs or genres tend to improve your mood and reduce pain, and which do not
- Engage in active listening by deliberately focusing mindfully on the music—note the changes in tempo, pay attention to the lyrics, try to discern the various instruments playing
- Use music both when in pain, and also preemptively—*before* your pain spikes or mood worsens—by creating a daily routine of listening for a predetermined amount of time
- If the music moves you, move your body!
- Bring your favorite music to physical therapy sessions to help reduce or prevent pain and distress related to PT

Aromatherapy

Aromatherapy is more than simply smelling something pleasant. It involves the distillation of essential oils from the leaves, peel, or other parts of plants for the broad purpose of enhancing well-being. Aromatherapy oils can then be delivered via the skin, your sense of smell, or orally. The molecules from essential oils travel from the nose to the olfactory bulb in the brain and then on to the limbic system, the areas of the brain that process emotions and memories.

Two structures in the limbic system, the amygdala and the hippocampus, are considered particularly important in the processing of aromas. The amygdala is a key area for processing emotions, and the hippocampus is involved in the formation of and ability to retrieve memories. The involvement of these brain structures in your sense of smell is why something as simple as smelling a particular laundry detergent or perfume can trigger thoughts of a beloved family member or former flame.

ALERT

Although technically some essential oils can be used orally, you should not add them to foods, beverages, or otherwise ingest them unless under the guidance of a skilled aromatherapist and with clearance from your physician. In addition, as a general rule, dilute essential oils properly before applying to the skin.

Similarly, you may pass a restaurant or bakery and the smell might temporarily transport you back in time to a cherished grandmother making your favorite dish or home-baked bread. Your association to these memories will determine the emotion that the smell generates. So, if you smell a familiar perfume you might experience a boost in mood even before you realize that this particular scent is the same one worn by your Great-Aunt Sophie. Passing the bakery might temporarily transport you back in time both to a cherished grandmother making your favorite pound cake and a feeling of being cared for.

Aromatherapy and Pain

Dr. Jane Buckle, a well-known researcher in aromatherapy, has speculated that lavandula angustifolia (true lavender) essential oil may have a similar effect on the amygdala to that of diazepam (Valium). Lavender oil is commonly used topically for pain relief and to induce feelings of relaxation. Relatedly, aromas that are specifically relaxing, such as rose, bergamot, and chamomile oils, and those that are considered more stimulating, such as lemon, peppermint, basil, and sweet orange oil, may help with pain because of their potential ability to improve mood or decrease feelings of stress.

It is also probable that some of the healing impact of aromatherapy is linked to its so often being paired with touch. As you are aware, pleasant touch and feeling relaxed both close the pain gate. More recent research has found that essential oils that are either applied to the skin or inhaled do in fact enter the bloodstream. As such, they also result in measurable and fairly rapid psychological effects.

FACT

Aromatherapy is considered to be one of the fastest-growing CAM therapies used by nurses, but its use is much less common among physicians. Aromatherapy can be used to enhance relaxation in the physically well, medically ill, and those at the end of life.

Although aromatherapy is still considered outside the realm of medically accepted therapies, clients' interest in this area has grown substantially over the past few decades. Most of those who use aromas for healing tend to do so as part of a whole-person approach to healthcare, rather than as a stand-alone treatment. When applied thoughtfully, aromas may be incorporated into more "mainstream" healthcare practices with good results.

What the Science Says about Aromatherapy

Research related to the impact of scents, particularly essential oils, on mood has increased since the 1970s. Specifically, there have been several studies on the use of essential oils, such as lavender, rose, and other pleasant aromas, to reduce stress. Lavender in particular has been shown to reduce self-reports of stress, and in some preliminary research was associated with increased peripheral blood flow (an effect associated with relaxation) and a decrease in blood pressure, as well as positive changes in heart rate variability. In another trial, peppermint and lavender essential oils were associated with increased accuracy while proofreading.

The calming benefits of pleasant aromas many not be limited to essential oils, however. In at least two studies, coconut scent has been associated with decreased startle response, whereas an unpleasant scent (Limburger cheese) was associated with an increased startle response. A more recent study suggested that exposure to pleasant scent (also coconut) may blunt the body's response to performing a stressful task and also enhance recovery after the stressor has stopped. It is important to note that most of these studies have had challenges with regard to their design, including having small numbers of people in the trials. Nonetheless, the results are thought provoking and may make intuitive sense to those who have experienced benefits from aromatherapy.

FACT

According to AromaWeb.com, many factors affect the price of aromatherapy oils. These include the rarity of the plant from which the oil is distilled, how much oil is produced by the plant, and the quality standards of the distiller.

Studies of aromatherapy in those who have dementia have preliminarily found that lavender and lemon balm oils reduced agitation, insomnia, wandering, and social withdrawal. Other studies with dementia patients found that a mix of multiple essential oils was linked to a reduction in disturbed behavior and reductions in psychiatric medications. A study with sage oil found a reduction in behavioral symptoms in patients with Alzheimer's. Other research has found improved memory with the use of rosemary oil and increased contentment with rosemary and lavender.

Lavender has been linked to improved sleep and reduced use of sedative medication in patients with dementia. Chamomile oil has also been associated with improved sleep. Both of these oils have been linked to reduced anxiety in patients with dementia.

Aroma in Psychotherapy

How might aromatherapy be relevant to the practice of psychotherapy? Pleasant aromas can be paired with relaxation training, such as diaphragmatic breathing, mindfulness practice, hypnotherapy, and biofeedback. Doing so may link the experience of relaxation with the scent sufficiently so that in the future, exposure to the scent alone may be enough to elicit the relaxation response. In cognitive-behavioral therapy, this pairing is referred to as "associative learning" or "higher-order conditioning," and the goal is for the scent to trigger the same response as the biofeedback, breathing, or meditation does, eventually on its own.

Aromas can also easily be used in at-home formal and informal mindfulness practice to facilitate "taking in" the present moment via smell. Examples include experiencing fully the aromas associated with eating, drinking, or walking in nature, as well as taking in the scent of the dish detergent when washing the dishes, and the like. Thus, being mindfully present can be "aromatherapeutic" or at least "aroma-aware"—even without deliberately introducing a specific scent.

FACT

Earl Grey tea is made of black tea leaves to which a very small amount of bergamot oil has been added. Therefore, when you sip a cup of antioxidant-rich Earl Grey tea, you are also having an "aromatherapeutic" experience.

With regard to aromatherapy, at-home use of pleasant aroma can also be as simple as adding a few drops of an essential oil to a hand or body lotion or hair conditioner, buying natural laundry or cleaning products that feature relaxing or invigorating essential oils, chewing a stick of peppermint gum when proofreading a term paper, or mindfully sipping a cup of fragrant tea.

Guidelines for Use

Aromatherapy oils appear to have significant anecdotal reports of benefits, and there is some research finding evidence to support these claims. It is important to treat essential oils with caution, however. Proper use typically means appropriately diluting essential oils in a carrier oil such as sweet almond oil or jojoba oil. Some oils, such as peppermint, should never be applied directly to the skin. And you should not take any oils orally without consulting with your physician and a trained aromatherapist. In addition, be aware of potential allergies to aromatherapy products; place undiluted oils on a tissue or another object to smell them rather than applying directly to the skin, and educate yourself about the properties associated with different oils before using.

With regard to regulation, the FDA classifies aromatherapy oils as a cosmetic, a drug, or both, depending on how the product is marketed. For example, if an aromatherapy product is marketed for treating or preventing a disease, the FDA considers this a drug claim, and the product will be regulated as such. For more information about the regulation of aromatherapy products, visit *www.fda.gov*.

For More Information about Aromatherapy

As stated previously, a variety of oils are associated with stress-reducing or relaxing benefits, including lavender, rose, chamomile, and bergamot, among others. Oils that are considered uplifting include grapefruit, lemon, lemongrass, and sweet orange oil. Oils like peppermint, eucalyptus, and rosemary are invigorating.

AromaWeb.com features information about dozens of different essential oils, as well as a large number of free aromatherapy recipes, articles, and more. Again, if you are hoping to use aromatherapy to address a specific concern, seek out a trained aromatherapist and discuss any potential remedies with your medical team to reduce the chance of negative interactions between essential oils and medications.

The National Association for Holistic Aromatherapy provides information about the recommended curricula for aromatherapy education, as well as a list of approved training programs and a searchable database of aromatherapists. For more information about issues related to aromatherapy, including links to recent research, issues related to safety, and more, visit *www.NAHA.org*.

Recipes

You can find recipes on sites like Aromaweb.com, and you can also buy pre-packaged blends from companies like Aura Cacia. Experiment and see which aromatherapy oils and combinations you like best.

Calming blend:

Add the following oils to a clean, airtight, dark glass container: 1 ounce of sweet almond or jojoba oil, 3 drops of sweet orange oil, and 5 drops of lavender. Swirl to mix. This mixture is properly diluted, so you can use for massage or put a few drops on a tissue near your bed before going to sleep. Apply any time you desire additional calm. You can find 2-ounce dropper bottles online or in your nearest health food store. Alternatively, you can use the previously mentioned ratio and add this plus one tablespoon of dried lavender to one pound of sea salts, adjusting the amount of lavender and oils to your preference. Mix thoroughly and store in airtight jars. Add a few tablespoons of the scented salts to your bath water.

Blend for stress relief:

Add the following to 1 ounce of sweet almond or jojoba oil: 4 drops of bergamot oil, 2 drops of rose geranium oil, and 5 drops of lavender oil. Mix and apply externally or to a tissue or cloth, or use to make a bath salt mixture.

You can also create single-note oils by adding a few drops of your favorites to 1 ounce of a carrier oil. Try neroli, rosemary, or balsam fir for an earthy, grounding scent; lavender or rose to help you relax; and lemon, bergamot, or rose geranium for a quick "pick-me-up." Remember that less is more. Start with two or three drops at first and add more little by little.

Finally, you can make aromatherapy sachets by drying your own herbs, including mint, lavender, oregano, rosemary, or thyme, etc., and combining them by what smells good to you. When in doubt, follow your nose!

CHAPTER 17

Spirituality

Spirituality is at once both universal and deeply personal. For some, spirituality is synonymous with religiosity, or formal involvement with an organized religion. Spirituality may also be less traditionally defined, representing a feeling of connectedness with something greater than oneself. Regardless of the definition used, it's worth knowing that religious coping is among the most popular CAM therapies in general, and frequently used by those in pain. Feeling connected to a religious community or the divine may help you find meaning and cope better despite pain.

Religious, Spiritual, Both, or Neither?

Until fairly recent times, religion and spirituality were considered to be undeniably linked, or even one and the same. Today, most people report some religious affiliation, but a growing number report being "spiritual but not religious." Essentially, this description refers to having no formal religious affiliation, but still feeling a connection to something greater than oneself, whether "the divine," "God," "the universe," "nature," or something else that feels personally meaningful.

To further complicate matters, there are still other people who report an affiliation to the religions they were raised in, but may not regularly attend services at a church, synagogue, mosque, or temple. And undoubtedly, there are those who are religiously observant but do not feel any sense of connection to the divine. And for still others, the concept of spirituality may not feel personally relevant at all.

FACT

A 2012 Pew Research Center polling found that one-fifth of the U.S. public, and a third of adults under thirty, are religiously unaffiliated. In the last five years, the unaffiliated have increased from just over 15 percent to just under 20 percent of all U.S. adults.

For the purposes of simplicity, religiosity and spirituality will be used interchangeably in this chapter, with the understanding that there are many ways in which someone may interpret either concept for himself. As you read on, allow the words spiritual and religious to mean whatever feels most comfortable and right for you.

Pain versus Suffering

You have likely heard the saying, "Pain is inevitable; suffering is optional." At first, this statement may appear to dismiss how challenging it can be to sit with pain, but the message could be one of the most helpful in enhancing your ability to cope. You already know quite a lot about pain as a mind-body experience involving your brain, nervous system, emotions, thoughts, and behaviors. Many times people take for granted that pain necessarily involves suffering; a way of understanding suffering, however, is that it is like an additional layer of something unpleasant or undesirable—whether self-pity, fear, worry, anger, judgment, etc.—that one overlays onto the pain experience itself. Very often, this process feels automatic, and the distress associated with pain becomes conflated, or made one and the same, with pain. Yet, pain and suffering are *not* synonymous and *do not* need to accompany each other.

Catastrophizing truly captures the "amping up" of the distress and awfulness of the pain experience. Thoughts like, "This can't be happening to me," "I can't bear this," "Things will never be okay," and "I can't live like this" are understandable reactions to the shock and dismay of developing chronic pain. But as you now know, catastrophizing has been shown to increase pain severity and decrease coping. Catastrophizing also undoubtedly contributes to suffering and gets in the way of *active coping*, or making changes that could help you live a life that has meaning for you. Without a sense of personal meaning, it can be much more difficult to find a reason to take care of a body in pain, or ride out the times when you feel anxiety, sadness, or grief about the changes associated with being in pain.

FACT

According to the Pew Research Center Survey, 65 percent of the U.S. general public identifies themselves as religious. Another 18 percent say they are not religious, but are spiritual—and 44 percent of those in this latter group pray daily. For more information, visit *www.pewresearch.org*.

Grief, Pain, and Coping

Even if your pain disorder is not life threatening, the loss of the body you once had can trigger profound grief akin to losing a loved one. Dr. Elisabeth Kübler-Ross, in her book *On Death and Dying*, outlined five stages of grief that she observed to be universal. Although Dr. Kübler-Ross initially based these stages on observing people who were dealing with a terminal illness, *any* significant life change can trigger feelings of grief.

The stages of grief are:

1. *Denial*—in which one deals with the shock of something by negating or denying the reality of the situation. This is a common reaction to the shock of a significant medical diagnosis and the changes that are associated with it. Common thoughts are, "This can't be happening" and "It's just not real."

2. *Anger*—which typically emerges as the denial wears off and the unfairness or distress of the situation hits home. This anger may be directed at the self, if there is a feeling that something you did led to this situation (whether or not that is true). Anger can also be directed at loved ones, or at the doctor who made the diagnosis. Your anger might also be more generalized and diffuse, such as when you feel angry at the world, or at others whose bodies are well. Common angry thoughts are, "This is totally unfair!" "This should not be happening to me!" and "A just God would not allow this to happen!" Anger and the other stages may also activate thoughts and feelings of envy such as "Why are they okay when I am not?"

3. *Bargaining*—which represents the very common behavior of promising something in return for something else. Bargaining may look like, "Dear God, if You will make this go away, I promise I will do XYZ." Bargaining can alternatingly instill brief hope and increase feelings of hopelessness when the situation fails to change (or when there is no divine intervention on your behalf).

4. *Depression*—which sets in as it becomes undeniably clear that the situation will not change. "Why bother?" "There's no hope," and "My life is over" are thoughts characteristic of depression.

5. *Acceptance*—which involves intellectually and emotionally acknowledging the reality of the situation as it is. Acceptance facilitates a clear understanding, without resistance, of what one can change versus what one cannot change. Acceptance involves agreeing to do what you can, but otherwise choosing to sit with the situation rather than directing energy toward a goal that will not be realized (e.g., accepting the loss of a limb rather than raging against that loss).

You have almost certainly experienced most or all of these stages since your diagnosis, and as you live with pain. You may also find at times, especially as your body changes, that you return to an earlier stage for a period of time.

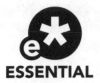

ESSENTIAL

Remember that your friends, family, or partner will *also* go through their own versions of the stages of grief because of their concern for you—whether or not their concern or worry are obvious. It is impossible to care about another without also experiencing distress at that person's difficulties.

Making Meaning As a Way of Coping

Spirituality can serve as a path to making meaning out of your life experiences, including pain and grief. There may be many times when you experience emotions, bodily sensations, or other changes in your life that feel as though they are too much to bear. Having a connection to something greater than yourself, whether a community of other people with whom you have something in common, or a connection that is religious in nature, can reinforce for you that you are not alone in your struggles. Connections with others and with the divine can remind you that your life has meaning and that you are important and have intrinsic worth even though your body and your life are different from what they were.

"Default Tools"

The challenge for many is that in a time of personal crisis it is easiest to reach for the ways of coping that are especially familiar or that you believe will be easiest, most effective, and most comforting in the moment. Sometimes the temptation is to reach for something comforting but unhealthy, such as smoking, consuming alcohol, overeating, misusing medication or taking street drugs, and the like. You will know when your coping tool is problematic by how you feel about your choice or yourself later on, when the "desirable effects" of the tool have worn off. If your tool of choice leaves you feeling guilty, ashamed, anxious, self-critical, or depressed, this is a sign that your coping strategy is not really beneficial and may even be harmful.

As you reflect on how your current coping strategy ultimately affects you, try to simply sit with and observe any uncomfortable thoughts and feelings that come up. What you learn in these moments can help you re-examine what truly would feel both helpful and most respectful of you—the person you are now, as well as the person you strive to be. This type of reflection can be a vital step in the process of making meaning.

Exercise

Take some time to reflect on and answer the following questions. They will help you get a sense of how you cope currently, and how you make meaning of your life as it is now, even with pain.

- When I feel stressed, I tend to:

_____

- When I use this tool (do for each item listed here), in the short term I feel:

_____

- A while after using this tool, my body feels:

_____

- A while after using this tool, my mind feels:

_____

- A while after using this tool, my thoughts and feelings about myself are:

_____

- Before I was in pain, I thought my purpose in life was:

_____

- Before I was in pain, my self-esteem was:

_____

- Currently, I feel my purpose in life is:

_____

- Currently, my self-esteem is:

_____

- Ideally, how would I like to view myself and my purpose in life?

_____

- In order to feel good about myself and my purpose in life, what (other than my pain) would need to change?

_____

After filling in these answers, think about how your responses fit with your personal spirituality or the teachings of your particular faith. If it feels difficult to find purpose or meaning in your life since developing pain, consider speaking with your clergy person, a friend you trust, or a qualified mental health professional.

Meaning making could also be thought of as a search for personal significance and purpose. Engaging in this process of self-examination can help you know at a deep level that you are here for a reason, even if you are not yet sure exactly what that means for you. Seeking meaning in your life helps you remember that even when things are difficult, painful, or feel like too much to bear, there may be something positive you can take from the experience.

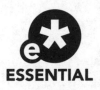

ESSENTIAL

Making meaning out of the life you have is *not* the same thing as saying you would choose to be in pain or experience suffering. But finding meaning in your life can help you make the suffering part of pain optional.

What the Science Says about Religiosity and Health

In recent years, there has been increasing research into the relationship between religion/spirituality and health. With regard to the impact of religiosity on pain and health, there is no definitive answer as of yet. Some studies show a positive impact of religiosity or spiritual connection, and some have found a negative effect (i.e., worse pain, mood, or functioning).

About half the studies found that religious involvement is linked to having fewer health problems and reduced risk of dying prematurely, while many others found no effect of religion on health. Some studies have even found that religiosity was linked to worse outcomes. These conflicting results can make it difficult to determine what, if any, effect religious involvement might have on your health. There are some factors that may explain the conflicting results.

Positive versus Negative Religious Coping

One possible reason for the lack of a clear relationship between religion and health is that someone can be religious but have difficulty making meaning of or coming to terms with pain. For example, *positive religious coping* might lead you to conclude that in each moment you are doing the best you can to cope with pain and that the rest is in God's hands. And while you might believe that God is ultimately in control, you may also understand that you can and should be proactive in managing your health. Another type of positive religious coping would be to decide that despite pain and the challenges that come with it, your pain condition inspires you to help others with a similar physical issue. In essence, you can still have a clear sense of purpose, even with pain.

Negative religious coping, although it may lead you to pray more, tends to reflect a greater degree of depression, hopelessness, resignation, or anxiety. You can be vulnerable to negative religious coping regardless of how religious you consider yourself. Examples of negative religious coping are attributing your pain to God punishing you, believing that your pain is evidence of inherent unworthiness or sinfulness, feeling God has abandoned you, or avoiding taking an active role in your health because you assume you will be healed if and only if this is the will of the divine.

As you can see, although both positive and negative religious coping are ways of relying on one's faith to understand and make meaning of personal difficulty, positive religious coping emphasizes being an active agent in your pain management and in your life in general. It also focuses on making what you can of the life and body you have now. An additional benefit of positive religious coping is that it may help you see yourself as having become stronger because of the challenges you have faced. Positive religious coping has been linked to having better interpersonal relationships, being more compassionate with others, and taking the perspective that life is precious despite one's difficulties. Not surprisingly, negative religious coping has been linked to greater depression.

Other Factors That Complicate the Picture

The social nature of human beings means that people live in and must come to terms with the values and beliefs of the many groups to which they belong. For example, you are an individual with your own likes and dislikes, understanding of yourself, your world, and the choices you make. Yet, you are also part of a family (whether or not the relationships are close ones).

Furthermore, you are part of an ethnic culture, national culture, live within a neighborhood, and perhaps also identify yourself as part of a particular political group. Your gender and sexuality also link you to others who share these traits. On top of this, you are part of a religious or spiritual culture—whether you consider yourself very religious, "spiritual but not religious," or not religious or spiritual at all.

Each layer of culture or identification can be a source of support or conflict for you. If you are part of a marginalized group, or feel persecuted or misunderstood in some way, whether for your religion, culture, economic status, country of origin, gender, or sexuality, this will undoubtedly increase your stress and create internal conflict. This tension may also generate questions about how a just God could allow injustice or suffering, or leave you feeling isolated or at odds with one of your identified groups. As a result, you may pray for assistance or as a way to cope (indicating some degree of religiosity), but the stress may nevertheless negatively affect your well-being. Such a situation can possibly explain the relationship between high levels of religiosity and poor physical or mental health.

FACT

Neuroscientist Dr. Andrew Newberg and his colleagues have examined how meditation and prayer affected the brains of both Buddhist meditators and Catholic nuns. They found that both meditation and prayer increased brain activity related to attention and concentration, and created a feeling of timelessness. Verbally oriented prayer increased activation in language areas. For more information on Dr. Newberg's work, visit AndrewNewberg.com.

Another factor that complicates the research into religiosity and health is that many religious people understandably object to the idea that human beings could presume to understand or influence the will of God. It will probably never be known why some people appear to "benefit" from spiritual or religious practices (i.e., decrease symptoms or improve health), and some "don't." Again, this illustrates the challenges inherent in studying the health effects of religiosity, or coming to a firm conclusion about whether it is generally healthful.

All of this aside, the bottom line is that if spiritual practices or affiliation feel important to you, affirm your worth as a human being, and bring you comfort, *these are reasons enough to continue engaging in them*. Connecting with a spiritual or even a meditative community can provide an invaluable source of social support and help keep catastrophizing in check. Ideally, your spiritual or religious involvement should remind you that you have worth and your life has meaning—despite pain or illness.

Cassandra, Suffering, and Liberation

Cassandra had experienced repeated abuse during childhood that left her with both severe chronic pain and posttraumatic stress. She was constantly anxious, had difficulty getting close to others, and had ongoing insomnia. Both Cassandra and her abuser had been part of a deeply religious community, and early on, Cassandra had been made to believe that her abuse and pain were the result of God's anger at her, or evidence of her inherent sinfulness. As a result, Cassandra felt she was unworthy of love or of having relief from pain.

Cassandra prayed daily that God would forgive her for whatever sin had led to her being in pain, but her distress, pain, and self-criticism persisted.

Although a part of her desired healing, and sought out treatment for her pain, a deeper part of Cassandra believed she deserved to suffer. None of the many medications she tried seemed to have any benefit, and Cassandra became more depressed as a result.

A turning point came when Cassandra began attending services at a new church, whose members believed in each person's inherent value, as well as in a loving God. Over time, with the support of a loving partner and in therapy, Cassandra began to challenge the assumption that her abuse, pain, and suffering were either deserved or proof of God's punishing her. "I've been thinking," she said, "that if God is loving, and teaches forgiveness, even if I *did* do something wrong, or am a sinner—and I mean, who isn't—it doesn't make sense that I'd be punished in this way."

In therapy, Cassandra learned about mindfulness, which helped her observe her fears, anxieties, sadness, and self-criticism without automatically taking these as "truth." Although Cassandra still struggled with mood and pain, she slowly began to view herself as an imperfect person who nevertheless had value at her core. Her distress and pain began to lessen.

Cassandra also learned self-hypnosis techniques for turning the volume down on pain, and releasing outdated ideas about herself. When she prayed, it was now to express gratitude for her newfound support, for whatever areas of her body felt comfortable, and to ask for further guidance and healing in whatever way was possible for her.

"I'm still in pain, and I still have challenges. And I'm still learning about what my relationship with God is all about. But I'm not suffering as much any more."

Ways to Enhance Spiritual Connection

There are a number of ways to connect with something greater than yourself, recognize what is good in the world and in your own life, and reap the benefits of doing so. The following are suggestions, but feel free to add your own ideas and practices to this list:

- Pray according to whatever custom resonates with you.
- Meditate. This practice stills the mind and calms the body. It's been said that prayer is talking to God; meditation is listening.

- Practice loving kindness.
- Perform acts of service.
- Be in nature.
- Be grateful. There is always something for which you can be grateful, even in times of difficulty.
- Release old hurts. Forgiveness can set you free from unhealthy attachments.
- Keep a journal of your meditations, insights, and those things that remind you of the divine in ordinary, everyday events. Note those things for which you are grateful.

Affirmations

Affirmations are present-tense, positive statements. Affirmations can help you change the unconscious messages that may have been contributing to your fear, worry, self-criticism, or catastrophizing. Creating affirmations is simple. Note the negative things you tell yourself, and write these down in a journal. Below each negative statement, write down a statement that reflects something in opposition to that sentiment. Make sure the affirmation is positive, and written in the present tense.

As an example, if a negative automatic thought arises, such as, "I am never going to be able to manage my pain," write this statement down. Writing it down makes the issue conscious, and therefore gives you a greater ability to create positive change. Underneath or next to this statement, you could write something like, "Each day, I am learning more about what my body needs, and feeling better." Another alternative statement could be, "Each day, I do the best I can, and am proud of my efforts." At the end of the week, on a separate page, write down all the positive affirmations you have created. Read each one to yourself out loud, morning and evening.

HealthJourneys.com features a large selection of audio programs that feature healing affirmations, as well as imagery or self-hypnosis, by area of interest. Among these are programs to enhance self-esteem, manage pain, create positive change, manage stress, and more. You can also listen to free samples of affirmations tracks to get a better sense of how to create statements that can help liberate you from limiting beliefs.

CHAPTER 18

Medical Marijuana

Marijuana has been used for medicinal purposes for approximately three thousand years. Medical marijuana remains a controversial and complicated topic in terms of the science, legal issues, and public perception. The Controlled Substances Act of 1970 placed marijuana in the Schedule I category, classifying it as having no medicinal value and high potential for abuse. More recently, however, patients, scientists, and politicians are reexamining whether marijuana has value for treating pain and other symptoms, particularly those that have not responded well to other interventions.

Marijuana as Medicine

As early as the mid-1800s, marijuana was introduced in the West as a potential therapy to ease pain, combat convulsions, help with sleep, and reduce muscle spasms. In the mid-1980s, the FDA approved a synthetic, oral form of marijuana's main psychoactive component, resulting in the drug dronabinol (brand name, Marinol).

Marinol was initially developed to treat chemotherapy-induced nausea and vomiting. Because of its effects on nausea and appetite, patients with HIV began using this drug. People with a variety of illnesses, such as cancer and chronic pain, have reported that although Marinol improves appetite, it may not necessarily result in needed weight gain—a benefit that is more commonly associated with using the entire marijuana plant.

Medical Marijuana

Medical marijuana (MM) refers to treating a disease or symptom with the whole, unprocessed marijuana plant or its basic extracts. At this writing, the FDA has not recognized or approved the marijuana plant as medicine. Yet for many in chronic pain, including some children with serious illnesses, MM may provide pain relief and other benefits without the side effects of many other medications. A number of myths and some stigma are attached to MM use, and both opponents and proponents feel strongly about whether MM should be available as medicine.

FACT

Scientists are conducting preclinical and clinical trials with marijuana and its extracts to treat numerous diseases and conditions. Two FDA-approved marijuana drugs are dronabinol and nabilone, both used to treat nausea and boost appetite.

The chemicals in marijuana that are thought to have therapeutic effects are called *cannabinoids*. You actually produce your own version of cannabinoids, called endocannabinoids, just as your body also produces its own type of opioids (called endogenous opioids). In addition, your body and brain have receptors that enable you to experience the effects of cannabinoids derived from MM.

The Legality of MM

In 2013, the FDA updated an inter-agency advisory regarding claims that smoked marijuana is medicine. In essence, the advisory states that marijuana continues to be listed in the class of substances that are most heavily restricted because marijuana has a high potential for abuse, has no currently accepted medical use in treatment in the United States, and has a lack of accepted safety for use under medical supervision. You can read the full text of this release on the FDA website (*www.fda.gov/NewsEvents/ Newsroom/PressAnnouncements/2006/ucm108643.htm*).

Despite the FDA and DEA's official position, since 1996, twenty-three states and Washington, DC, have passed laws allowing smoked marijuana to be used for a variety of medical conditions. For further information regarding the federal government's position on marijuana, visit *www.whitehouse.gov*.

The Pros of Legalizing of Medical Marijuana

As with most substances, and all medications, there are potential risks as well as benefits to MM. Proponents of MM have proposed that legalization would:

- Ensure a product that is standardized and quality-controlled
- Establish the therapeutic doses most likely to maximize benefit and reduce risks
- Control the production and sale of MM
- Make the public aware of technologies to reduce risks (vaporizers) and educate regarding proper MM use

There are a number of terms related to MM, and it can be challenging to remember these. You may wish to refer to the accompanying list as you read this chapter and other resources about MM.

Here are a few key terms related to marijuana:

- *THC (delta-9-tetrahydrocannabinol)*: This is the main psychoactive, or mind-altering chemical in MM. Psychoactive effects include the relaxation and euphoria associated with smoking or consuming marijuana. Undesirable psychoactive effects can include paranoia, depression, and less frequently, psychotic symptoms. THC may also decrease pain, inflammation (swelling and redness), and muscle control problems, such as those seen in epilepsy.
- *Cannabidiol or CBD*: CBD does not affect the mind or behavior. It may be useful in reducing pain and inflammation; controlling epileptic seizures, including in childhood epilepsy; and possibly even treating mental illness and addictions. CBD is thought to counteract the psychoactive effects of THC.
- *Cannabinoids*: These are chemicals related to THC. Other than THC, the marijuana plant contains more than 100 other cannabinoids. Both scientists and illegal manufacturers have produced many cannabinoids in the lab.
- *CB1*: This is one of two known cannabinoid receptors, and is located on neurons (nerve cells) in the brain and spinal cord.
- *CB2*: This is the other known type of cannabinoid receptor. CB2 is located primarily on immune cells, but they are also found in neurons that contain the brain chemical dopamine in the ventral tegmental area of the brain. This area is involved in both reward and drug addiction.
- *Endocannabinoids*: These are the body's own cannabinoids. They play a role in regulating pleasure, memory, thinking, concentration, body movement, awareness of time, appetite, pain, and the senses (taste, touch, smell, hearing, and sight).

Cannabis Research

What follows is necessarily a very brief overview of some of the MM research to date. In one example, because CB2 receptors are located in the body's immune cells, a 2003 study examined the impact of MM, either smoked or taken orally, on the immune response of HIV-positive patients. Receiving cannabinoids was not associated with negative effects on immune function, nor was it linked to interactions with participants' medications. In addition, the participants who received MM also gained significantly more weight (a desirable outcome) than those who did not receive MM.

The Missoula Chronic Clinical Cannabis Use Study examined the therapeutic benefits and adverse effects of prolonged use of medical marijuana in four seriously ill patients. This research was approved through the Compassionate Investigational New Drug program of the FDA. The researchers found that MM had several benefits. The side effects noted after long-term use were mild changes in lung function in two of the four patients. There were no significant negative effects noted, including on MRI scans of the brain, chest X-rays, neuropsychological tests, hormone and immunological tests, and clinical examinations.

Benefits observed in the patients in this study are summarized here. A woman with glaucoma and cataracts experienced improved intraocular pressure and sight, and reduced insomnia. A man with a genetic disorder causing abnormally formed or absent nails and kneecaps, kidney failure, and severe chronic pain that did not respond to other medications experienced less pain, fewer spasms, improved ability to walk, decreased nausea, and improved sleep. A man who had over 250 hereditary bony tumors, chronic pain, and limited analgesia from large doses of opioid pain medications experienced a pain reduction of five points (from 9/10 to 4/10). The fourth patient, a woman with multiple sclerosis who suffered from muscle spasms and optic nerve damage that impaired her vision, as well as anxiety, depression, nausea, and insomnia, experienced improvements in all these symptoms.

This study was extremely small and the results are not generalizable to the larger population of medically ill people. Yet, the findings are not without value because the study looked at the effects of long-term use on people who had multiple, serious, longstanding, and complex medical issues that had not responded well to other treatments.

FACT

According to the 2013 National Survey on Drug Use, marijuana use is widespread among adolescents and young adults. It is the most commonly used street drug in the United States, with approximately 20 million users per month.

The University of Washington's Alcohol and Drug Abuse Institute (ADAI) maintains a detailed and comprehensive website that addresses a number of issues related to marijuana use. Among these are summaries of the research, information about drug policy, findings related to adult and teen use, resources for parents, Spanish-language information, and more. Visit *http://learnaboutmarijuanawa.org*. The ADAI's summary regarding MM, and the chronic pain research, states that the cannabinoids in MM are similar to the endocannabinoids produced by the human body and that they can alleviate pain that has not responded to traditional medical treatments. The website summarizes the research findings with regard to MM's benefits in those with multiple sclerosis, cancer, fibromyalgia, HIV, and neuropathic pain. Furthermore, because cannabidiol can inhibit THC's psychoactive effects, they state that MM is best tolerated when high levels of CBD are present.

In addition, similar to other proponents' statements about the benefits of MM, the ADAI's position is that MM is a relatively safe medication as compared to many prescription drugs for chronic pain, such as opioid pain medications.

Policy

The National Institute on Drug Abuse (NIDA) is a scientific rather than a policy-making agency. The data from NIDA research is likely to influence MM policy, however. Currently, NIDA's position is that the research data available suggests that THC and other cannabinoids may have potential in the treatment of pain, nausea, obesity, wasting disease, addiction, autoimmune disorders, and other conditions. NIDA is currently funding studies on the use of THC and CBD for the treatment of pain and addiction. Their research is also examining the antipsychotic effects of CBD, which may lead to new treatment options for people with schizophrenia.

NIDA concludes that to date, researchers have not conducted enough large-scale clinical trials that show that the benefits of the marijuana plant (as opposed to its cannabinoid ingredients) outweigh its risks in the patients it is meant to treat.

For more information about NIDA's current clinical trials, and to see if you are eligible to participate in any of them, visit *www.drugabuse.gov/clinical-trial/search*.

Compassionate Use

Several states have enacted laws to provide MM as "compassionate care." As an example, New York State enacted a Compassionate Use Law in June of 2014. This law will allow healthcare providers to recommend the medical use of marijuana under carefully controlled circumstances. Compassionate Care NY (*www.compassionatecareny.org*), a statewide group of patients, providers, and lawmakers worked with the Drug Policy Alliance (*www.drugpolicy.org*) to advocate for this legislation. The Drug Policy Alliance has information about the current drug laws in each state. You can visit their website for more information.

Risks of Medical Marijuana Use

A 2008 review of the MM research found that short-term use of MM use was linked to increased likelihood of non-serious side effects as compared to no treatment, with dizziness being the most common. The rate of serious adverse effects was the same in both the MM and control conditions (suggesting no additional risk from MM over no treatment). The most common serious adverse effects were relapse of multiple sclerosis, vomiting, and urinary tract infection.

ALERT

Marijuana users who carry a specific variant of the AKT1 gene are at increased risk of developing psychosis. One study found that the risk of psychosis for those with this genetic variant was seven times higher for daily marijuana users compared with infrequent- or non-users.

In March 2013, Dr. Nora Volkow, the director of NIDA, issued a statement about a large-scale study of marijuana that found that heavy use in the teen years was associated with significant declines in IQ scores (an average of eight points). Dr. Volkow said this finding is consistent with those from animal studies. To read her statement in its entirety, visit *www.drugabuse.gov/about-nida/directors-page/messages-director/2012/09/marijuanas-lasting-effects-brain.%5BAU*.

ALERT

The amount of THC can vary in edible marijuana products, including homemade ones. In addition, they can be harmful to children and pets so keep these products away from both!

More research is being done to understand the effects of regular or heavy marijuana use on adolescent brain development. The risks do not appear to be the same for adults, yet marijuana is not risk-free. For a more thorough discussion of the known and potential risks of long-term, heavy, or early marijuana use, visit *www.drugabuse.gov*. Some of the risks associated with marijuana use are outlined here:

- Marijuana consumed in foods results in a delayed effect as compared to smoking, because the drug must pass through the digestive system. This delay may cause users to inadvertently consume more THC and other chemicals than they intend to.
- Although marijuana frequently induces pleasant feelings, such as relaxation and euphoria, it can also cause feelings of anxiety, fear, distrust, or panic. Large doses can result in temporary symptoms of psychosis, such as hallucinations, delusions, and feelings of depersonalization (the loss of a sense of personal identity).
- THC can alter the function of several areas of the brain and result in impaired thinking and ability to learn and perform complicated tasks, as well as changes in balance, coordination, and reaction time.
- Marijuana's potency has increased over the past few decades, with current samples having approximately three times the amount of THC as samples from the 1990s.
- A number of studies have found a link between marijuana use and increased risk of mental illnesses, including psychotic illness, depression, and anxiety. This risk is most likely greater in people who have a genetic or other biological vulnerability to these illnesses.
- Marijuana has been linked to what is referred to as "amotivational syndrome." This syndrome is characterized by a diminished or absent drive to engage in productive or typically rewarding activities.
- Cannabis can be addictive.

- Marijuana can be dangerous for people with cardiopulmonary disease, respiratory insufficiency, or liver or kidney disease.
- Marijuana may be harmful to fetal development.

To summarize, the topic of whether or not marijuana should be an FDA-approved medicine is a complex one to address, and it is beyond the scope of this chapter to fully do the issue justice. Both opponents and proponents have made impassioned arguments. Furthermore, the scientific literature to date has shed light on both the potential risks and the medical benefits of marijuana, but much more research needs to be conducted before there will be a clear consensus. If your pain, nausea, vomiting, or other symptoms have not responded sufficiently to approved drugs, and you are wondering about the legality, risks, and potential benefits of MM, speak with your healthcare provider. You may also wish to consult the Internet resources mentioned here for more up-to-date information about the state of MM legislation in your area.

Your Integrative Pain Management Plan

By now, you probably know more than you ever imagined you would about CAM therapies and an integrative approach for managing pain. In fact, there is a good chance that you know more about integrative treatments than many of your conventional medical providers. Please feel free to share this book or the resources contained within with the members of your health-care team. The more you and your providers—CAM and conventional— can work together, the better the odds that you will feel supported and your pain will be as well managed as possible.

Over time, you will probably wish to refer back to the chapters on the therapies you wish to try, and it's recommended that you also create a sepa-rate notebook to keep track of what is most helpful, as well as what is not. Here are some suggestions and tips to help you make healthy changes and achieve a greater sense of well-being.

Put your plan into action. Starting with broad goals, decide what you would like to see change. For example, do you hope to increase your flexibil-ity, muscular strength, or energy levels? Will your plan include modifications to your diet, or exercise? Do you hope to increase your social interactions with others? Are you hoping to reconnect with the spiritual side of your life?

Make a list of these goals. Periodically revisit the list to see if there is any-thing you would like to add or change.

_____

_____

Now, determine a priority order for the goals listed. Write them down, in order. Your chance of success is probably going to be greater if you give yourself adequate time to make each change sequentially, one at a time. At most, try to take on no more than two or three changes at a time, at least ini-tially. Which goal do you want to address first? Second? Third?

_____

_____

Take each goal listed, and break it down into smaller, manageable steps.

For example, if you hope to improve your diet, what will this look like? Will it involve reducing or eliminating nightshade vegetables if you suffer from arthritis? If your goal is improved fitness, will it mean increasing the type, intensity, or duration of exercise? If you hope to expand your support network, or enhance feelings of spiritual connectedness, perhaps it will mean contacting members of a religious or spiritual organization near you. Be concrete and specific with regard to the steps you will take.

_____

_____

Now take a look at your calendar. An old-fashioned paper calendar often works best for this purpose. Being realistic, decide by when you hope to achieve your larger goal. Write it down on the date you choose as your completion date. Then, take the individual steps you listed previously and spread them out, giving each step the appropriate amount of time for you to reach it. If need be, check with others, perhaps your physical therapist, dietitian, or a trusted friend, to make sure the time you have allotted for achieving each step is realistic.

If you like, write down the "due dates" for each phase of your process so you can easily refer back to them.

_____

_____

Enlisting some "cheerleaders" during this process will enhance your chances of success and your enjoyment during this process. Note potential cheerleaders, coaches, or other supporters. Some of these may be professionals, such as a dietitian to help you make significant dietary changes, or your doctor to help you determine how much weight is safe for you to lose each week.

You may find that you also want to include others with a similar diagnosis on this team, such as someone you meet through a pain support group. Your family, friends, or partner may also serve as important cheerleaders. And a clergy member or friend from your religious community may help you remember that your worth is intrinsic—certainly more than the sum of your accomplishments or how your body is functioning—and that you are never alone.

List potential or current members of your support network. Revisit and update this list as your network expands or changes. Write something down even if you begin with one person, a health professional, or a beloved pet.

_____

_____

On a regular basis, look back on what you have accomplished with regard to learning and making healthy changes. Periodically remember where you were one month or one year ago. Acknowledge what you have achieved, without using the word "but . . . " even if it feels like there is still more work to be done. If you notice the temptation to say, "I have accomplished X, but it's not Y yet," stop yourself. Say instead, "I have accomplished X, and I am grateful and proud of this fact. I am now working toward accomplishing Y."

TIPS TO REMEMBER

- Whether your self-care plan ultimately winds up being more CAM, or largely conventional, remember to continue monitoring and treating any chronic conditions, including keeping up with any necessary diagnostic workups.
- Do keep a pain and mood diary, especially when you add or subtract a therapy—whether CAM or conventional—from your routine. This will help you more accurately assess if something is working, and if so, how well. Too often people discard a therapy that is helping because it's hard for them to realize a smaller or more gradual, but still significant, change in pain intensity or coping.
- Related, remember, small changes still count! A two-point difference on a ten-point scale (a change of 20 percent) is considered clinically meaningful.
- Anything you *do* creates change. The results of some of your actions will take longer to notice than others, but by making a conscious choice for change and then taking steps to that effect, you put yourself back in the

driver's seat. *And that is far more empowering than waiting for things to change or resenting where you are now.*

- Remember, too, that *avoiding taking action is also a type of choice.* You ultimately decide the stance or action you will take and what you will or will not do. Either way, give yourself the gift of taking the reins.
- Sometimes you will choose to focus on relaxation or pacing—which may feel like "non-action." But these are valid, health-supportive, and conscious choices and are quite different from refusing to do anything at all. Thus, these types of non-doing also put you in the driver's seat.
- Schedule self-care activities into your calendar, just as you would any other important appointments.
- Pacing is essential to good self-care!
- *Commit to living, right now*—whatever that means for you—rather than waiting to start living until your pain dissipates or your health changes. Making this commitment may be one of the most powerful and healing things that you do.
- Release the habit of comparing yourself to others, including your former self.
- Remember, ups and downs are completely normal and to be expected. Use your energy for other things than focusing on temporary challenges or setbacks. *You are in it for the long haul.*
- Practice gratitude. Appreciate what's good about your body, your life, and who you are—in this very moment.
- Find out what gives your life meaning. Nurture that part of you or aspect of your life.
- When your pain and distress become amplified and threaten to overwhelm you, practice moving your awareness outside you to the world around you. Note what is wonderful and miraculous in the everyday—a child laughing, a flower opening, the seasons changing. And when you notice the difficulties others face, allow this to activate your compassion. When you can be of service to another, do this, even if the gesture seems small to you. Helping others is an unexpected but powerful tool for self-healing and makes the world a better place.
- Remember, *this moment* is the only one you ever truly have. Be in "the gift of the present."
- Forgive yourself for being imperfect. Perfection is simply an illusion, and just gets in the way of healing.

Resources

As you continue on your journey of pain management and healthy change, you may wish to learn more about the topics covered in this book. Following is a variety of resources you can consult for more information. Some of them are links to professional organizations for CAM and conventional providers. Others will provide you with everything from general information to the latest research about a particular therapy.

Academy of Integrative Health & Medicine
https://aihm.org

American Chronic Pain Association
www.theacpa.org

American Academy of Medical Acupuncture
www.medicalacupuncture.org

American Academy of Pain Medicine
www.aapainmanage.org

American Association of Naturopathic Physicians
www.naturopathic.org

American Board of Medical Specialties
www.abms.org

American Board of Pain Medicine
www.abpm.org

American Chiropractic Association
www.acatoday.org/index

Academy of Nutrition and Dietetics (formerly the American Dietetic Association)
www.eatright.org

American Massage Therapy Association
www.amtamassage.org

American Osteopathic Association
www.osteopathic.org/Pages/default.aspx

American Pain Society
http://americanpainsociety.org

American Psychological Association
www.APA.org

American Society of Clinical Hypnosis
www.asch.net

Appcrawlr (to research apps relevant to a particular task or goal)
http://appcrawlr.com

AromaWeb (aromatherapy information)
http://aromaweb.com

Association for Applied Psychophysiology and Biofeedback
www.aapb.org

Beck Institute for Cognitive Behavior Therapy
www.beckinstitute.org

Biofeedback Certification International Alliance
www.BCIA.org

Centers for Disease Control and Prevention (Physical Activity Guidelines)
www.cdc.gov/physicalactivity/everyone/guidelines/

Center for Mindfulness
www.umassmed.edu/cfm/

The Center for Reiki Research
http://centerforreikiresearch.org

The Certification Board for Music Therapists
www.cbmt.org

ClinicalTrials.gov (to find a clinical trial)
https://clinicaltrials.gov

Consumerlab.com (information about dietary supplement quality and research)
www.consumerlab.com

Drug Policy Alliance (advocacy organization supporting legalization of medical marijuana)
www.drugpolicy.org

Friends Health Connection (support and education for those who have a chronic illness)
www.FriendsHealthConnection.org

Guided Mindfulness Meditation Practices with Jon Kabat-Zinn
www.mindfulnesscds.com

GoodTherapy.org (information about psychotherapy and provider referral website)
www.goodtherapy.org

Healing Touch Program
www.healingtouchprogram.com

Health Journeys (guided imagery and hypnosis audio programs)
www.healthjourneys.com

International Association for the Study of Pain
www.iasp-pain.org

The Monroe Institute (Hemi-Sync Audio Programs)
www.monroeinstitute.org

National Association for Cognitive Behavioral Therapists
www.nacbt.org

The National Association for Holistic Aromatherapy
www.naha.org

National Center for Complementary and Integrative Health (formerly NCCAM)
http://NCCIH.NIH.gov

The National Certification Commission for Acupuncture and Oriental Medicine
www.nccaom.org

National Institute on Drug Abuse
www.drugabuse.gov

National Institutes of Health, Office of Dietary Supplements
https://ods.od.nih.gov/Health_Information/ Dietary_Reference_Intakes.aspx

Pew Research Center
www.pewresearch.org

Psychology Today Online
www.psychologytoday.com

PubMed
www.ncbi.nlm.nih.gov/pubmed/

The Reiki Alliance
www.reikialliance.com

R. J. Buckle Associates (Dr. Jane Buckle's page on aromatherapy)
www.rjbuckle.com

Sounds True (audio programs)
www.soundstrue.com

Therapeutic Touch International Association
http://therapeutic-touch.org

Tara Brach's website (free mindfulness audios)
www.tarabrach.com/audioarchives-guided-meditations.html

The University of Washington, Alcohol and Drug Abuse Institute
http://learnaboutmarijuanawa.org

UCLA Mindful Awareness Research Center (free mindfulness audios)
http://marc.ucla.edu/body.cfm?id=22

WebMD
www.WebMD.com

Index